M767

Successful Veterinary Nurse Training

Medway Campus

Class No: 636.089 YAT

Return on or before the date last stamped below:

For renewals phone 01634 383044

Pocket Practice Guides

Series Editors: Carl Gorman BVSc MRCVS and Sue Gorman BVSc MRCVS

Clients, Pets and Vets
Communication and management
Carl Gorman

Finance, Employment and Wealth for Vets
Second Edition
Keith Dickinson

The Veterinary Support Team
Maggie Shilcock

Premises for Vets
Designing the Veterinary Habitat
Jim Wishart

Interviewing and Recruiting Veterinary Staff
Maggie Shilcock

Prosperity after Practice
Retirement planning for vets
Mike Nelson

Successful Veterinary Nurse Training
Jo Yates

Pocket Practice Guides

Successful Veterinary Nurse Training

Jo Yates
DipAVN(Surgical) VN

Illustrated by Hayley Albrecht

Threshold Press

First published 2004 by
Threshold Press Ltd, 152 Craven Road
Newbury, Berks RG14 5NR
Phone: 01635-230272 Fax: 01635-44804
email: publish@threshold-press.co.uk
www.threshold-press.co.uk

ISBN 1-903152-14-3

Typeset by Threshold Press Ltd
Printed in England by Biddles Ltd, Kings Lynn

The Illustrator
Hayley Albrecht obtained an honours degree in silversmithing at Loughborough
in 1996 and has worked in this field and as an artist ever since. She was an award
winner at the Society of Equestrian Artists' annual exhibition at Christie's in
2000.

Contents

Glossary of Terms and Abbreviations

Assessment	Measurement of how effectively a student has learned, usually measured against stated learning outcomes
Awarding Body	A professional body that oversees and sets the standards for a particular qualification. They, in turn, are answerable to QCA. For example, the RCVS is the awarding body for veterinary nursing
BVNA	British Veterinary Nursing Association
CPD	Continuing Professional Development
GCSE	General Certificate of Secondary Education
HE	Higher Education
IV	Internal Verifier
Lantra	The Sector Skills Council for Environmental and Land-based Sector Training
MCQ	Multiple-Choice Question. This is the form taken by the VN qualification examinations
NVQ	National Vocational Qualification Work-based evidence collected to meet national occupational standards
Occupational Standards	Specific written units of criteria, used to measure students' competence
QCA	Qualifications and Curriculum Authority
RCVS	Royal College of Veterinary Surgeons
SVQ	Scottish Vocational Qualifications
TP	Training Practice
VNAC	Veterinary Nursing Approved Centre
VRQ	Vocationally Related Qualification

List of Figures

Acknowledgements

My grateful thanks go to Lynn Rose, as without her support and managerial skills quite literally none of this would have happened. Thanks also to those vets and nurses in the East Midlands who continue to work with me at Bottle Green Training to educate and train their student nurses.

The author and publishers are grateful to RCVS for permission to reproduce the guidance notes and log sheet and to Lantra for permission to reprint the Units and elements of the NVQ standards

Lastly I need to thank my family and friends, with special reference to one morning over 16 years ago and the incident of the 'matching bin liners' – Jeannie, I have done it!

1

Choosing a Veterinary Nursing Training Scheme

To be perfect is to change often

ANY VETERINARY PRACTICE OR INDIVIDUAL who is considering working within the veterinary nursing training scheme needs an insight into its background to make informed decisions relating to their individual needs. This chapter looks at the brief history of veterinary nurse training and outlines the current approaches to training members of the nursing team. Educational ideals, qualifications and concepts are in a constant state of flux. However, the use of a work-based format as the central method of veterinary nurse training has persisted relatively unchanged. This is a comfort as, after all, the main purpose and outcome of the RCVS training scheme is essentially a qualified veterinary nurse.

The story so far

It was not until the early 1960s that a recognised training and examination programme was established for veterinary nurses. In 1961 the scheme that was the beginning of the present training system was inaugurated by the RCVS. In those early days the award title was Registered Animal Nursing Auxiliary. At that time, the title of 'nurse' was jealously guarded by the Royal College of Nursing, so the term 'nurse' was restricted to those qualified in human nursing. It was not until 1984, after much professional wrangling, that the term 'veterinary nurse' became an accepted title.

Whatever the title, the training scheme for veterinary nurses has changed little over the intervening years. It essentially still involves a two-year course of tuition that runs alongside workplace training and experience. In those days the practices supporting trainees were known as approved training centres (ATCs) and, like today's training practices, they had to meet certain criteria set down by the RCVS. These criteria worked to ensure that each student was, as far as possible, working in a standardised environment and experiencing a similar clinical caseload. Written examinations were taken at the end of each year. The work-based or practical skills were identified and competences recorded in a 'practical book'. These practical skills were also examined at the end of each year.

Today the scheme has evolved to include a portfolio of evidence designed to offer evidence of the students' practical skills assessed and certificated by a trained and named assessor. The development of a set of industry-specific occupational standards enables assessors to standardise decision about competence. In using the occupational standards set by the RCVS, it is possible to ensure each student achieves the skills necessary to function as a veterinary nurse. The end-of-year examinations are still present, along with one final set of practical exams. The trainee nurses must still register with the RCVS and the practices that wish to support trainees still need to be approved by the RCVS against specified criteria. Today such practices are known as training practices (TPs).

This type of apprenticeship scheme suits the very practical nature of the veterinary nurse's role. Nursing skills are many and varied and learning takes place through 'doing': this may explain the unchanged nature of the scheme over the years. For example, it is impossible to learn the skill of catheter placement while sitting in a classroom, just as good patient care is difficult to learn from a text. The practical elements of veterinary nursing need to be learnt and practiced in the workplace.

Today there are various routes of training and education to enable the individual to gain the title of veterinary nurse. They all still demand core practical experience that has to be gained in a training practice which has been inspected and approved through the RCVS Veterinary Nursing Scheme.

The Veterinary Nurse Certificate

1   Work-based training by NVQ/VRQ

National Vocational Qualifications (NVQs) or Vocationally Related Qualifications (VRQs) are the current educational packages that surround the Veterinary Nursing certificate. They are called NVQs in England and Wales and SVQs in Scotland (for Scottish Vocational Qualifications). As with many things 'educational', the precise details of exactly how the standard veterinary nurse qualification is packaged will always depend upon the current political and financial climate.

Whatever we choose to call the current and 'in vogue' route for veterinary nurse training there is no escaping the vocational nature of the job. The continuing practical requirement for special skills is met by an apprenticeship-style training scheme. This method of training forms the successful mainstay of veterinary nursing.

National Vocational Qualifications were introduced into the veterinary nurse scheme back in 1998. This system involves the use of occupational standards set by the awarding body (the RCVS) that are to be used by suitably qualified workplace assessors to measure levels of competence and successful achievement of each trainee nurse within a workplace. The occupational standards identify the essential skill areas necessary for an individual to attain in order to become a veterinary nurse.

A portfolio has been designed by the RCVS as a series of log sheets that are to be completed in an almost diary-like format. This attempts to give a structure or framework within which the trainee can fully demonstrate the key competencies that are relevant to veterinary nursing. The training practice is expected to provide clinical training opportunities to support the student nurse through the training period – usually a minimum of two years.

In conjunction with the experiences of the workplace, the student attends a lecture-based course of academic learning following a theory syllabus set by the RCVS. This theory course may be attended on a day-release or block-release system, usually in a further education college. The particular approach taken is often dictated by the geographical position of the veterinary practice in relation to the college course provider. The course is divided into two years or levels. The first year of study is Level 2, followed by a multiple-choice external examination, and the second year is Level 3, followed again by an external examination including a practical element. The external examinations are conducted by the RCVS as the awarding body for the Veterinary Nursing Certificate.

As with all things educational, the Veterinary Nursing Certificate has to have a value within the market place of education. This is the value of the Veterinary Nursing Certificate as a commodity to the individual, not only within the vocational area of veterinary medicine but also as an educational qualification that may be transferred to another training course in an alternative occupational area. Many courses are becoming modularised so that credits may be accumulated and transferred or taken forward for use at a later stage if education is continued.

Veterinary nurse training, however small the number of students, cannot escape the attention of the regulators and the qualification is being forced to conform to the current ideals and concepts in education and training. Apparently we are all members of a learning society, hence the changes that seem to be a constant part of the veterinary nurse training scheme. There have been quite a few changes but thankfully they all appear to be variations on a theme – that of work-based vocational apprenticeship training. Long may it be preserved.

The ideal of a learning society with all these inter-related levels of qualifications also extends to encompass and promote a framework for Continuing Professional Development or CPD as it is called within the veterinary industry.

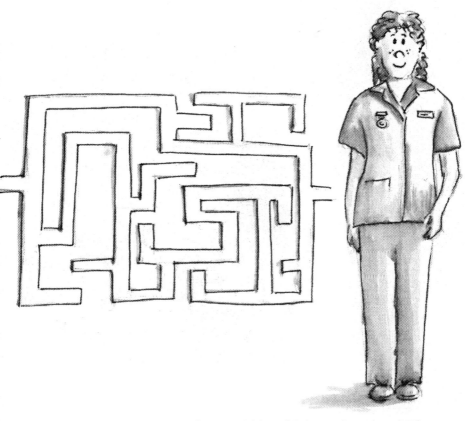

2   Veterinary Nurse Certificate within a higher education (HE)
     qualification

It is now possible to follow the veterinary nursing course as an
integral part of a three or four-year degree course. An increasing
number of colleges offer science-based degree courses that link into
the veterinary nursing syllabus. This route obviously takes longer
to complete but still involves time out in practice as blocks of work
experience and professional examinations still have to be passed.

The best route?

This is a question that needs to be answered by the training practice
and also the individual potential student. We will look at each route,
the respective entry requirements of the courses and the vital issue
of funding.

1 Work-based training

Essentially both routes contain the element of work-based training. Individual practices must consider what type of practice they are, and how they can incorporate and manage a training scheme within their working ethos. Training has to be built into the business-and-development plan for each veterinary business. Not every practice can commit to the responsibility for training nurses at certificate level. They should not feel any less professional for admitting this; it is in no way a reflection of their clinical skills. It is important to be very aware that training veterinary nurses is not for everyone.

Each training practice needs to have an assessor who will take on the responsibility of making the decisions about the practical competence of the student nurse. Each assessor (a qualified vet or veterinary nurse) is normally able to support two trainees at a time. This restriction is set to ensure that the assessor is not overloaded with the necessary time and effort that each student requires. The RCVS recommends that each student receives three hours of tutorial/teaching support, within the practice, every week.

It is so important to be aware of the realistic number of working hours that you need to invest in each student. At this point the training practice should consider which type of student they can support for work-based training: either the employed-apprentice type of student or the temporary or part-time HE student.

❑ There is potentially less disruption with a 'permanent' (if apprenticed) member of the team. Their assessments and evidence for log sheets can be collected at more flexible and regular intervals during the busy working schedule.

❑ A 'temporary' member of staff provided from the pool of HE students may prove more convenient for a shorter time period with less restrictions for long-term employment.

❑ Some practices may regard HE students as a free or cheap pair of hands. Be warned that nothing in this world is for free. These students still require time and support equal to those working through the more traditional apprentice route.

❑ Training nurses by the HE route may prove an excellent way of 'choosing' the correct personality to join the practice team once they are qualified. You can perhaps think of the training period as an extended type of interview.

❏ Each assessor and student will need to be internally verified by their college/VNAC (Veterinary Nursing Approved Centre) to ensure standardisation of work-based assessments. This will potentially involve quite a few practice visits if the training practice is supporting students from different sources. Each centre may use a different system for paperwork.

❏ For more detailed information on internal verification and VNACs see Chapter 7. In brief: internal verifiers are provided to support the assessor in practice (who will be a senior nurse or vet or similarly qualified person). All training practices belong to a VNAC. The VNACs use internal verifiers to visit the training practices to check that standards are being maintained and that the students are being correctly supported in their work-based skill training.

❏ With the apprenticeship route, it is easier for the practice to stay informed and involved with the training in theory that the student is receiving in the classroom. This gives the advantage of being able to link work-based skills with practical application and collection of evidence for the portfolio.

❏ In taking on HE students the practice will limit the number of employed trainees they can support. For example, to support two HE students the assessor's time will be fully allocated, thus precluding the employment of a full-time trainee.

❏ Some practices have reported that HE students appear to be more motivated in their collection of evidence. However, this comment is very specific to the individual personality and one can come across difficult-to-motivate individuals at any educational level.

❏ Most practices have a complicated rota system, especially when covering for holidays, etc. A student who is working on a day-release apprentice system may prove less of a problem with regard to staffing levels.

2 Entry requirements

The choice of training route may to some extent be decided for the individual by the educational entry requirements for each type of course.

At certificate level (NVQ/VRQ) using the day/block-release system, the student needs to be educated to GCSE level and hold five certificates of grade C or above, to include English and Maths or Science.

There are other exam awards that will meet the above criteria and a full list of equivalencies is available from the RCVS Veterinary Nursing Department (see Useful Addresses at end of book). One of the most popular and successful routes of entry is the Animal Nursing Assistant certificate which is operated by the BVNA (British Veterinary Nursing Association) in conjunction with the Awarding Body Consortium. This examination course has no restrictions on entry and usually takes a year to complete; the courses are taught by further education colleges and agricultural colleges.

The HE or degree route requires the usual A level examination passes and each college sets its own requirements. Mature students may be selected on different criteria set by the individual colleges.

The increase in the number and variety of training courses for veterinary nursing is designed to meet the differing needs of both individuals and industry, working within government educational policies. All routes to the veterinary nurse certificate incorporate the acquisition by the individual of an NVQ certificate in conjunction with the successful completion of examinations, set against a syllabus of the theoretical knowledge.

The number of veterinary nursing students is to some extent limited by the number of training practices and hence the number of trainee jobs available. The smaller practices usually can only support one trainee, whereas the larger hospitals or group practices are sufficiently staffed and organised to train two or three. The number of trained assessors employed controls the number of students that each practice can support at the recommended ratio of one assessor to two students.

These facts need to be taken into account if the individual student is looking for 'temporary' placement in order to gain the necessary practical experience required as part of a higher educational course. Host practices may be difficult to find if they already carry their full quota of trainees.

3 Funding and finance

The cost of training is an important consideration for any small business. Veterinary practices have become particularly aware of this cost, following the introduction of the NVQ system and the necessity for trained assessors in the workplace. Each training practice must be supported by internal verification. Thus internal verification fees may be an additional annual cost for all training practices, regardless of the type of student they support.

HE students are self-funded and therefore are only expensive in terms of support and training time. This is almost a hidden cost and not always fully appreciated by practices. The long-term financial implications for individuals undertaking HE for a probable four-year period need to be understood.

Practical training undertaken in a 'host' practice may pay a minimum wage but this is only for 70 weeks. The rest of the time spent in full-time HE.

The financial rewards that are usually expected by postgraduates do not easily translate in the veterinary small-business world, especially if the veterinary nurse wishes to undertake a general nursing role. Unfortunately, the veterinary nursing profession is not well paid. There are of course other, possibly more lucrative, career pathways to be followed within the veterinary industry for those graduates who hold a science degree combined with veterinary nursing.

For the more traditional and vocational route to the veterinary nurse certificate, paid employment is undertaken over the two-year training period. The employer is usually assisted by a government training agency which directly funds the cost of the two-year taught college course (in England, this is the local Learning and Skills Council, but funding conditions may vary from area to area).

Most students who train by this route will find that on completion of training their employment status is naturally continued within the veterinary practice that worked so hard to support them in their training. These students will have the security of a full-time job and, if they are fortunate, they will not have an educational loan to repay.

Student profile 1   Alison

Alison passed her Animal Nursing Assistant certificate last summer, allowing her to meet the entry requirements for the RCVS VN scheme. Alison did not enjoy school and she left education at the first opportunity. She has been employed in a veterinary practice for four years and is a valued member of staff. The practice was registered as a TP and Alison was encouraged to gain an official qualification. She is now thoroughly enjoying her day-release college course and has worked hard to complete her portfolio for her NVQ at Level 2. Her confidence in the workplace has increased and she is looking forward to further responsibilities when she has achieved VN status.

The following appendix is an example taken from Module 7 of the portfolio, Medical Nursing and Fluid Therapy. The guidance notes are followed by a log which has been assessed by an assessor using the Occupational Standards for VN8. These documents are copyright RCVS and are reprinted with their kind permission.

Appendix to Chapter 1

Module 7 – Medical Nursing and Fluid Therapy Guidance Notes for Students and Assessors

Introduction

This module is designed to cover the following Veterinary Nursing Occupational Standards:

Unit VN8 - Administer veterinary medical nursing care to animals

EVIDENCE REQUIREMENT

Log Sheets Titles	Number of Log Sheets Required
7a Medical Nursing	6
- Expanded case reports	2
7b Fluid Therapy	3

If you follow the guidance for each type of log sheet, the evidence requirements for NVQ Level 3 — unit VN8 should be covered. However reference should be made to the relevant Occupational Standards to ensure appropriate aspects are assessed and to help direct appropriate assessor questioning.

GUIDANCE NOTES FOR LOG SHEET 7a

7a   Medical Nursing   6 logs

You are required to complete a log sheet for **six** medical cases in which you have played an active role in the nursing of each animal. The cases chosen should cover a broad spectrum of medical cases and reflect a range of body systems. Your practical involvement will need to focus on procedures associated with the diagnosis of the medical condition, the administration of treatments and monitoring.

You may cross-reference these cases to other modules within this level if this is appropriate. Your cases should include **three different** species i.e. dogs, cats and one other small pet/exotic. Reference can also be made to the medical nursing section of the objective syllabus to help you chose the appropriate cases, however here are some suggestions:

- Diarrhoeic patients
- Obese patients
- Pregnancy
- Parturition
- Pancreatic insufficiency
- Infectious/contagious diseases
- Diabetes mellitus
- Renal failure
- Dermatological conditions
- Cardiac conditions
- Poisoning

Expanded Case Reports

Two of the six medical log sheets should be expanded into **approximately** 1000 word case reports, in which you are expected to demonstrate your knowledge and understanding of the condition, treatment and nursing management. You must also include a copy of the patient monitoring record for each of these two cases.

Headings for Case Reports

Case reference
Case details
Presenting problem and history
Preliminary clinical finding
Diagnostic procedures and testing
Treatment and nursing
Ongoing management of condition
Outcome and case evaluation

7b   Fluid therapy   3 logs

You are required to complete log sheets for **three** cases which have received fluid therapy. You will need to have played an *active role in the administration and maintenance of the fluid therapy and the monitoring of the animal.

(* placement of Intravenous catheter by the candidate is expected in at least one of the cases.)

You should cover both cats and dogs. You should cover **three** of the following different types of fluid therapy:

- Crystalloids
- Colloids
- Blood
- Oral rehydration.

You are encouraged to cross-reference the fluid logs to the medical cases used within this module. However it is acceptable to cross-reference to any other cases used in this level. It must be made clear which cases the fluid therapy logs relate to.

NB: For each log sheet you are required to include a copy of the patient-monitoring chart used to record and monitor the fluid therapy.

Log Sheet 7b – Fluid Management

Student Veterinary Nurse's Name		Jo Yates	VN Enrolment number			E621422
1 Case Details	Breed	Domestic short hair	Age	10 yrs	Sex	M(n)
	Species	Feline	Weight	5kg		

2 Case No identification

30104 – Clint

3 Reason for administering fluid

Prolonged period of vomiting and diarrhoea – 48 hours

4 Type of fluid selected: *According to veterinary surgeon's instructions*

Crystalloid – Hartmann's solution (Lactated Ringers Solution)

5 Reason for choice of fluid and route of administration

Replacement of mixed electrolyte and water losses

Correction of metabolic acidosis (Diarrhoea and prolonged vomiting)

I.V. route – cephalic vein.

6 Equipment and supplies: *State what was selected and how it was prepared in order to administer the fluids.*

Giving set, Burette and 500 mls of Hartmann's. Bag of fluid warmed to body temp.

Date and contents of bag checked.

I.V. catheter 22 gauge, tape, dressings, skin preparation (chlorhexadine, surgical spirit), Hepflush to flush catheter when placed.

Fluid bag, burette, giving set connected aseptically and fluid run through, leaving no air bubbles in line.

I.V. catheter aseptically placed in right cephalic vein. Taped in place. Hepflush to maintain patency of catheter.

Assessor's Comments
VN 8.1
VN 8.1 Student aware of patient monitoring (pc 6).
Supporting evidence of chart included.
VN 8.3 (pc 3) Monitoring regime.
VN 8.1 (pc 3)
VN 8.2
Student-placed catheter aseptical.
Correct disposal of waste observed.
VN 8.1 (pc 8)

7 Fluid therapy plan: a) Estimated total fluid deficit & b) Rate of administration (include ml per hour and drip rate *Show how volume (a) and rates (b) were calculated*	
First 24 hrs losses replaced – guess at 8% dehydration (no on-going losses) and maintenance (8%) loss to be given over 6 hours. Maintenance over 18 hrs.	

Loss $= \dfrac{8 \times 5 \text{ kgs}}{100} = 400$ mls plus Maintenance over 18 hrs $= 50 \times 5 = 250$ mls

$\dfrac{400}{6} = 66$ mls/hr over 6 hrs

$\dfrac{66}{60} = 1$ ml/min

$\dfrac{250}{18} = 13.8$ mls/hr

$\dfrac{13.8}{60} = 0.23$ mls/min

Burette gives 60 drops/ml
$= 60 \times 1 = 60$ drops/min

Burette gives 60 drops/ml
$= 60 \times 0.23 = 13$ drops/min

8 Summary of fluid therapy plan: any revisions to the initial plan

No further losses, so the next 24 hrs continued at maintenance rate. Patient started to drink and recovered well.

Maintenance $= \dfrac{250 \text{ mls}}{24} = 10.4$ mls/hr

$\dfrac{10.4}{60} = 0.17$ mls/min

Burette gives 60 drops/ml $= 60 \times 0.17 = 10$ drops/minute

9 Monitoring the animal: a) Monitoring of administration, urine output, vital signs etc. & animal's progress. b) A recording chart/record used by you to monitor this animal must be attached.	
Patient seems quite bright, even though showing clinical signs of dehydration. Skin testing etc 8% was guessed at. TPR and catheter checked every 20 minutes during the first 6 hours of replacement therapy. CRT and mm checked and improvement seen after 4 hours of therapy. (No lab tests were performed due to client's restricted costs.) Urine output was measured and patient watched for further V & D. None apparent. See detailed chart for recordings and readings. Oral fluids were introduced after 6 hours. Food was offered that evening.	*VN 8.1 Vet informed of patient's condition. (pc1 thru 7) VN 8.2 Feeding introduced as requested (pc 3, 4 & 6)*
Date(s) to include: full timescale range, if appropriate......30/1/04–1/2/04	

Student's comments and signature

Comments

Although this patient was showing signs of quite severe dehydration, he was quite bright and responsive. No further episodes of vomiting or diarrhoea were seen, so no adjustments were made to the initial plan. A burette was used to further control the amount of liquid infused and to guard against 'over-infusion' in a relatively small patient. The catheter was actually removed after 30 hours as the patient was eating and drinking normally.

The evidence in this log sheet is a true account of the case/procedures described and of my involvement therein. The work undertaken in compiling the log is my own.

Student Veterinary Nurse's Signature..............

Assessor's statement

The procedures and details recorded within this log sheet have been observed by myself / a witness* (Witness's name...............) and have been carried out correctly and competently. (*Please delete)

Comments

The student is extremely competent in this area and demonstrated good clinical nursing skills. In order to meet the standards, detailed discussion was carried out concerning Health and Safety issues and disposal of waste (VN 8.1, pc 8,9).
Good reflection on use of burette. The next patient type should be canine in order to meet the scope for this unit. A different type of fluid needs to be chosen. There is still a need for an exotic case; however, this may need to be covered by oral questions.

Assessor's signature..............   Assessor's name..............

Assessor's qualifications..............   Date...2/2/04...

2

Teaching and Learning in the Workplace

Human history is more and more a race between
education and catastrophe

UNFORTUNATELY THE NVQ SYSTEM, when introduced, was
rather heavily 'skewed' towards the process of assessment and
the attainment of competence. Little attention was given to the
process of actual teaching and learning that must take place. As
training practices rushed to acquire a qualified assessor, the necessary skills and understanding required for effective clinical teaching
were in some cases overlooked.

The named assessor within practice is also often the individual
who is responsible for training and teaching the student. Very few
have received any formal input on how to maximise the learning
opportunities for their trainees. The following chapter deals with a
little of the theory of teaching and learning that may prove useful
to anyone undertaking the responsibility of training a student nurse
in the workplace.

As with most subjects, a few concepts have to be mastered to
inform and support meaningful practice.

Concepts of education and training

Education
Education is a planned, contrived and purposeful learning opportunity with the development of a knowledge base and understanding
that leads eventually to 'altered' behaviour. Education generally

takes place in an institutional establishment: a school, college or classroom base, etc.

Training

Training prepares someone to perform a task or role, typically within a workplace. This involves both instruction and practice in order for the individual to reach a particular level of competence. Achievement of competence may be linked to change of behaviour and it is arguable that a certain level of understanding is required to undertake the task correctly. So it can be seen that some educational and training processes and outcomes are linked.

Figure 1   Educational and training processes and outcomes are linked

Education and training are best pictured as sitting at the opposite ends of a spectrum. Education is the more general, broader activity; with training being a more restricted and specific activity.

Figure 2   The education and training continuum

Education   Training

$\longleftarrow\!\longrightarrow$

increasing in breadth and depth   increasing in specificity

The boundaries between education and training are not clear-cut. Education is at the academic or 'knowledge' end of the spectrum, with training and practical 'doing' at the opposite end. Consequently, most workplace skills fall within the middle range, with strong affinity for practical application and training. This is particularly true of vocational jobs such as those in the service industries. Clearly the right framework for teaching and training for a vocational job should be designed to maximise the likelihood of an appropriate and successful outcome.

The vocational nature of veterinary nursing lends itself to the training concept – hence the requirement for work-based and practical experience of skills as an integral part of any learning programme undertaken to gain the Veterinary Nursing Certificate.

Learning

Learning is about change. Learning is usually brought about intentionally – for instance, when we attend a course or read an informative text, perhaps in a veterinary journal. Learning is relatively permanent. It is the developing of a new skill, understanding a scientific law or changing an attitude. Some learning can take place without planning and intention – for example, veterinary staff soon learn what their feline patients are indicating with that gently twitching tail tip and flattened ears. Life is one long learning experience.

There are two models of learning – traditional and modern. The modern approach is driven by educational theory that is based in psychology and the study of behaviour.

As trainers in the workplace we need to know how people behave under certain circumstances, so that we can optimise their learning through the provision of conditions that make the process as easy as possible. If a teacher controls the learners' educational experiences too much, they limit the amount of personal growth that can occur. Nursing education will then churn out clones of the profession, who do not question what they see and who neither trust or know themselves.

Recent work on learning indicates that

❑ Learning is active, not the passive receipt of knowledge and skills
❑ Learning is personal and individual
❑ Learning is voluntary, we need to do it ourselves.

Figure 3	Learning models compared
Traditional/input model	**Modern/action model**
Passive	Active
Reception	Search
Fill a deficit	Seek for satisfaction
Responsive to outside stimulus	Initiated by need
Keywords may be 'give', 'impart'	Keywords: 'discover', 'create'
Transfer of knowledge and skill	Problem-solving
Need for a teacher	Self-learning

Types of learning

It is important to take a holistic approach to training if a reasonably balanced and useful individual – in this instance, specifically a veterinary nurse – is the expected outcome. Within the concept of learning, three separate areas or domains have been identified.

Psychomotor domain

This is the skill area concerned with physical dexterity: for example, in giving an injection or placing a suture. Both of the tasks do need knowledge but, predominantly, they are physical skills and require practice. The individual observes and imitates the skill in the first instance and then moves through the precision stage to being able to complete the skill or task automatically.

Cognitive domain

This is the thinking-skill area: the 'how' and 'why' of knowing and knowledge. For example: why is this drug being administered and what might be the side effects, if any? How will this wound heal? The cognitive domain works from the simple level of recall of information through to that of application with evaluation and finally arriving at the highest level within this domain – that of decision-making.

Affective domain

This is the one group that is often neglected within the academic and educational sphere. This deals with the feelings and emotions – the skill of anticipating a client's needs, or indeed a patient's needs within a specific nursing care plan. By looking at these models and concepts we can reach a clearer understanding of the aims and objectives of work-based learning.

Experiential learning

This chapter is concerned with the process of learning within the workplace and a key part of this is the idea of 'experiential learning'. In this approach, learning is presented as a continuous process grounded in experience. Learning is a holistic process, with learning from practical experience an excellent example – clinical nursing practice perhaps?

This concept of the learning process translates directly to the veterinary nursing scheme and the collection of evidence for the portfolio. The log sheets provide evidence of the student's learning, in this case very definitely grounded in experience. The content of the logs is then assessed and evaluated by the assessor and by the student. From this evaluation comes a reflection on the student's actions and on what has been learnt.

This reflection will then drive the student to collect the next piece of evidence. By using the occupational standards and the portfolio format, the trainee nurse should progress towards the goal of that final veterinary nurse qualification. Learning by doing is a practical aid to developing nursing skills.

Figure 4	The experiential learning cycle in veterinary nursing

Using Level 3 – Fluid Therapy skill as an example

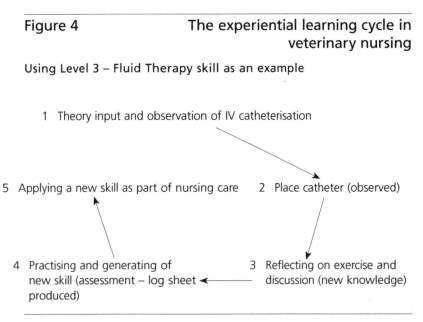

1 Theory input and observation of IV catheterisation

5 Applying a new skill as part of nursing care

2 Place catheter (observed)

4 Practising and generating of new skill (assessment – log sheet produced)

3 Reflecting on exercise and discussion (new knowledge)

This idea moves away from the more traditional 'input' type of learning and towards the modern 'action' type of learning. By using this framework for learning, the student is placed at the centre of the process and becomes a direct participant rather than an observer on the periphery. The role of the training practice is to support and guide the student. Perhaps the title of assessor, for the specified individual working on behalf of the training practice, has the wrong overtones. This may explain the apparent over-emphasis on the assessment of outcomes rather than the training process itself. Maybe the title of 'mentor' would be more appropriate.

How we learn

Having contrasted the theories of learning, this is the moment to consider how people learn. We are all individuals and each person has their own preferred method of learning. By using their preferred method, learning can take place relatively easily and with greater meaning. This goes a little way to explain that, when external factors are consistent, one person learns and the other does not. Perhaps the learning opportunity provided by being 'pitched in at the deep end' with minimal guidance will suit one person but will not work for another individual, who prefers to be given information and ideas on how to do it before 'having a go'. Most people are unaware of their learning preferences and it is helpful for the tutor or trainer to understand how their student learns in order to facilitate effective learning.

There is much literature published on learning styles; however, four main styles have been identified.

❑ Activist

Activists enjoy the 'here and now' and are dominated by immediate and instant experience. They tend to revel in the short-term crisis.

❑ Reflector

This group likes to stand back and ponder on experience, even observing the experience from a different angle. They collect data and analyse before coming to any conclusion.

❑ Theorist

This type of learner enjoys principles, theories, models and system-

atic thinking. They are rational and logical.
❑ Pragmatist
They positively search out new ideas and schemes and take the first
opportunity to experiment.

It is interesting to note that these 'styles' tend to be reinforced as
the individual matures. Very often people gravitate towards careers
and workplace environments that are compatible with their preferred method of working. It will come as no surprise to realise that
veterinary nurses are often the same type of learner: they are the
activists and even the pragmatists. Be aware that often individuals
have more than one style, and of course there are always exceptions
to the rule.

It is always difficult to wade through the theory, especially educational theory, but it is important to have an understanding of some
of the issues and to gain an insight into where the portfolio and
workplace training is based.

Perhaps by being aware of the theories behind learning and
training, some of the 'difficulties' in the workplace training and
assessment scheme for veterinary nursing may be resolved or even
avoided. Of course, these principles can be applied to any workplace
training. For example, when a new piece of equipment or a new protocol is introduced in the clinic, qualified and experienced members
of staff will all have their own preffered learning style and the trick
is to deliver the input accordingly.

Clinical teaching

As mentioned at the beginning of this chapter, when it was introduced, the NVQ scheme appeared to training practices to emphasise
the process of assessing skills. This seemed to be at the expense of
the teaching and input of knowledge. A basic understanding of the
skills and requirements for successful clinical teaching is certainly
equally important.

It is important to focus on the process of a procedure as well
as the outcome. This is the 'how to do it' part. Nursing skills are
used in practice in the context of patient care. This means that the
nurse must be able to apply and adapt key nursing skills in a variety

of different circumstances. Very often this detail becomes lost as the competent individual becomes an experienced practitioner. The experienced individual may even develop short cuts that may appear to be 'poor' practice. However, these short cuts taken by an experienced professional may in certain circumstances be perfectly acceptable. It should be remembered that if these actions were taken by an inexperienced individual or novice there might be dire consequences. We all develop 'habits', but the policy of teaching a student in a clinical situation the correct rules and protocols for each procedure must be adhered to. It can be quite difficult to look at a specific skill and break the process and actions down into simple stages or steps in order to teach and demonstrate to a student.

Clinical teaching may involve 'unlearning' bad habits not just for the tutor but also for the team in the workplace. It is so important that the training practice, as a whole, takes on the responsibility of training a student veterinary nurse and it is not just left to one designated person. Having made the choice to become a training practice, many practices find their standards of veterinary practice are improved and the business actually becomes more efficient, providing a higher level of patient and client care.

Important points to be considered when undertaking clinical teaching

Planning and tutorials

Although it is possible to teach while working in practice, some skills will require time set aside for teaching – especially those more complex skills such as care and maintenance of a fluid line. Some theory is involved here, not to mention mathematical calculations to be mastered. The student will be attending a college course but some points still need reinforcement from time to time. As part of a training practice's responsibility, three hours of training needs to be given to each student every week. It is also useful to use planning and tutorial sessions to establish the level of the student's existing knowledge and skill in order to develop training and teaching sessions further.

Demonstration of the skill in its real context
This is essential for the student to be able to relate to the relevance of the skill as it may be only be practised out of context or as a simulation until a reasonable level of competency has been reached.

Identification of the key stages of the skill
It is quite a difficult task to break down a 'skill' into almost bite-sized chunks. Once this has been done a demonstration needs to be carried out, in slow time if possible, highlighting the key stages of the task.

Performance of skill by student under close guidance
Student to practice the skill under supervision gaining experience in a real context. At this stage the student should be able to reflect on successful progress and be prepared to undertake an assessment.

Assessment is planned and carried out in clinical practice
It is important for the assessor and the student to understand the link between the occupational standards and the assessment. The occupational standards outline the framework of necessary skills required to demonstrate competence.

They give a broad outline of the clinical skills that it is deemed necessary for veterinary nurses to acquire. The fine details are missing and this calls for professional input from an experienced member of the veterinary team. There are now a number of texts available with standardised clinical protocols that can be followed. These texts have been long-awaited, as in the past only American publications were available. 'Animal technicians' are the American para-professionals to the veterinary industry.

There is a common theme running through all the standards and indeed through all the practical tasks and skills for veterinary nursing. These generic points create an acronym – ASIA – which can be a good starting point or be used as as a framework for teaching specific skills.

A sepsis

S afety for both the operator and the patient

I dentification and use of equipment

A ccuracy of outcome.

Using the example of fluid therapy and the nursing skills that entails

A Aseptic technique for placement of catheter connection and maintenance of giving set

S Correct handling of patient

I Correct choice of catheter gauge, giving set

A Correct calculation of drip rate and accurate placement of catheter.

ASIA is relevant to all the identified skill areas: medical nursing, surgical nursing, laboratory and even radiography to name but a few. These areas are set out as units within the occupational standards for veterinary nursing.

And finally to assessment

Perhaps this next section will help to bring together the relevance of all the theory and the assessor's certificate.

The dictionary definition of assessment suggests 'action taken to put a value on something'. In educational and training terms assessment is about finding out about students' abilities, possibly measuring performance in a formal way.

Assessments may be

Formative

As the name suggests, this concerns informing of progress and level of attainment so far. Assessments used in the formative style also give direction and guidance to the learner by identifying areas of competency not yet reached. Put simply, formative assessment can tell us 'where to go next' – a process leading to an outcome.

Summative

This has to do with the final decision concerning the learning that has taken place. The examination is an example of this type of assessment in formal education. The final internal verification report on the veterinary nursing portfolio is another example of summative assessment.

Most assessments can be seen as having an element of both formative and summative, particularly when effective feedback is given. The skill of the assessor in a practice is to use the assessment as a learning opportunity, as a useful basis for further development.

This might go some way to explain why the assessor should receive some formal training and direction on how to assess and why they, in turn, should build a portfolio of evidence to be assessed to a standard as set by the A Units (the new style D Units). Unfortunately, the quality of training received by many assessors is variable and misunderstandings are common. Assessment, used meaningfully in the formative style, highlights the importance of setting aside time in the workplace routine for tutorials and planning.

Ultimately, the assessment process will underpin the achievement of competence by the student measured against the occupational standards. The assessor is responsible for ensuring that each trainee nurse has reached the standards set.

The assessor needs to be:

❏ Familiar with the principles of vocational training and able to interpret the occupational standards for veterinary nursing.
❏ Aware of the need to achieve the certificate of competence in assessing (A Units or the old D Units).
❏ Experienced in veterinary nursing or veterinary surgery.
❏ Able to support and guide the student through the training scheme, identifying gaps in achievement.
❏ The assessor also needs to be able to give constructive feedback, to be encouraging and motivational.
❏ Most important of all, the assessor must be interested in the student's progress.

Methods of assessment that can be easily used for assessing veterinary nursing students in the practice environment are:

Direct observation
This method makes use of naturally occurring evidence from the workplace performance. The student is operating within a whole work role rather than in isolation. It is a good form of continual assessment and often requires other forms of assessment to ensure consistency. The assessor needs to be trained to ensure quality assurance.

Questioning
This can be very useful for collecting evidence of a student's competence, and oral or written questions can be used. Oral questioning works well to establish the student's application of knowledge and skill to a range of circumstances, especially when linked to direct observation. Lines of questioning can be easily recorded on the log sheets for inclusion in the student's portfolio.

Specially set tasks or simulations
These may be used when it is apparent that not all of the range or scope of each unit will be naturally covered during the training period.

Portfolio log sheets
These can be completed as set by the RCVS, or may be written assignments or projects.

The assessment of the student veterinary nurse is an ongoing process. Therefore it is important to plan quite long term for the collection of all the necessary evidence as set out in the standards. It is also important to have the time set aside to negotiate changes to the plan or include further items if necessary. The assessment process is rather dynamic and will depend upon the student's ability and the occurrence of necessary clinical opportunities within the workplace.

Occupational standards

The occupational standards are divided into units that represent each skill area set for veterinary nursing. Each unit is made up of two or three elements that break down to statements of competence that must be met by each student. Evidence of this competence is presented by a portfolio of log sheets – written evidence of the student's work skills, related and referenced to the individual units of the standards.

In conclusion, it can be seen that the occupational standards play an integral part in workplace training. They can be used to identify and direct training and teaching plans, and also to guide and inform assessment decisions.

Assessor profile 1   Nigel

Nigel, a very busy veterinary surgeon working as a partner in a small animal practice, was reluctantly coerced into the role of assessor. He enjoyed the role of assessor but found that the time he was spending with the practice's two students did not make economic sense.

During the last round of staff appraisals, he managed to identify a senior nurse who would be able to take over the role of practice assessor. She has started her A unit training and already the student nurses have made better progress with their portfolios.

Nigel is still involved with the training as he has to support the new assessor and he also holds regular tutorials with the students. Other nurses within the team are showing an interest in assessor training and the practice manager is working to build assessor training into staff CPD plans.

3

The Responsibilities of a Training Practice

If you have knowledge let others light their candles at it

THERE ARE A NUMBER of different practice 'types' with a range from large hospital organisations to the small country one-vet practices. Any type of practice can successfully train their own student veterinary nurses providing they are committed as a team and working to a good clinical standard. Each training practice is required to undergo an inspection to establish their suitability and capability to support a student nurse for their work-based training.

Facilities for clinical practice

The RCVS is the awarding body for the Veterinary Nursing Certificate. Its role is to set a standard of essential physical resources that each training practice must have in order to train students. These requirements are set in order to ensure that all student veterinary nurses work in an environment that relates to their theoretical training and allows them to collect the necessary evidence for their portfolio.

For example, it is difficult to demonstrate working practice with a microscope if the practice does not possess one. The laboratory module is quite a significant section at Level 3 and skills in this area are also tested during the practical examinations. Inspection of practice premises has to be carried out before approval is given. This inspection will be ongoing throughout the training period to ensure that no major changes take place that may compromise the student's prospects.

It is often not possible for branch surgeries to meet these minimum standards, usually due to the very fact that they are branches. It would be expected that major procedures are transferred to the larger better-equipped surgery, and therefore it is not possible for branch surgeries to support a student veterinary nurse.

The Responsibilities of a Training Practice

Health and safety

The practice is required to demonstrate understanding and compliance with workplace laws. In a well-run small business this should not prove to be a problem; however, a lot of veterinary surgeons dislike paper work and this aspect of the veterinary business can be a little neglected and disorganised. This is the area of veterinary practice that generally benefits from the attention of a practice manager.

Training practices need to demonstrate that they regularly monitor health and safety. Evidence of this may be found in

❑ a written protocol for induction sessions for new employees
❑ local rules drawn up and prominently displayed in the relevant work areas
❑ standard operating procedures and protocols when carrying out procedures involving equipment, such as operating the biochemistry machine or using an X-ray machine
❑ logged training sessions for new staff and training sessions concerning the use of new pieces of equipment
❑ a log book of equipment servicing and repair.

Employment law

Details of employment regulations and employment law now form an integral part of an NVQ and any other vocationally related qualification. It is important that each individual understands their rights and responsibilities as an employee and equally the rights and responsibilities of their employer.

Everyone needs to be aware of details such as

❑ contracts of employment
❑ minimum wage
❑ maximum number of hours in a working week
❑ sickness pay
❑ maternity issues
❑ individual practice/business policy on holidays, overtime, notice etc.

Clinical caseload

It is necessary for a training practice to work with a good caseload so that the student has the opportunity to 'nurse' a variety of species and types of case. Their portfolio of evidence should demonstrate a good range of different nursing skills applied not just to the more traditional small animal pet, the cat and the dog, but to the smaller, wriggly, fluffy, squeaky and often 'biting' type of patient. Of course, it is now possible to follow the nurse training and complete with an equine certificate. The patients nursed for this portfolio of evidence have to be of a very different specification.

Some smaller practices can experience a problem with caseload. This can be overcome with a bit of organisation and good planning. One of the most common problems is the number of radiographic cases that could reasonably be expected during the student's training period. It is possible to arrange for a 'work experience' placement in a larger training establishment in order to practise the necessary skills and collect any missing evidence for the portfolio. This approach works surprisingly well for both the student and the practice. In the larger and busier environment, the student has the opportunity to pick up and practise different nursing skills and bring ideas and routines back to the home practice.

Practical experience in the laboratory can often be limited in one single veterinary clinic. However, again if the student is given the opportunity to carry out work experience in a laboratory environment, these extra skills can be practised to perfection and beyond.

Patient-care protocols

Each veterinary nurse student has to collect a portfolio of evidence of skills achieved within the workplace. This evidence is assessed to meet the national standards set by the RCVS. During the rather onerous training undertaken by assessors for their certificate of competence, assessors discover that there are various types of valid evidence that can be presented by the student.

Work-based product evidence is one such type of evidence. The collection of such evidence is actively requested by the portfolio instructions in each module. This work-based evidence takes the form of charts and paperwork used by the nurse to monitor and care for the patient. Hospital sheets, intensive care sheets and anaesthetic charts are all good examples. The training practice should already be using such records as part of their standard patient care.

If this type of record-keeping is a normal part of the nursing routine the student will be able to quickly collect enough evidence to meet the requirements of the occupational standards set for each module. The use of good detailed supporting evidence reduces the need to write excessive and often repetitive details on the individual log sheets. Good organisation of the nursing team is essential for any training practice.

All practices should be keeping hospital and anaesthetic charts, especially in view of the fact that we live and work in an increasingly litigious world, so that they have written evidence of the quality of care they provide.

Continuing professional development

It is important for the training practice to have a positive and active approach to continuing professional development (CPD) for all the team. Any veterinary business in our modern and increasingly information-orientated society needs to build CPD into its long-term development and business plans. Next to the clinical resources, the human resources of any business need to be developed and utilised to ensure successful growth. Any practice that does not actively take part in CPD should not consider itself suitable as a trainer of veterinary nurses.

Training a student veterinary nurse will involve the whole team – everyone will learn, not just the student. Skills, protocols and methods of working change, new information is constantly being made available and everyone needs to be kept up to date. With the advent of the internet and the globalisation of information, clients are much more informed and CPD is important from that aspect of the business, let alone for the staff-training benefits.

A bit of organisation is needed here, with a budget perhaps set for each individual. All this learning needs to be documented and recorded, unfortunately resulting in the generation of yet more paperwork. CPD is already an accepted part of the veterinary surgeon's professional status and increasingly it will become part of a listed veterinary nurse's status too.

Equipment and facilities to support training

A well-stocked library is a 'must' for any practice. A practice with training-practice status should have a good range of texts that are suitable to support a student at nurse level. Over the last few years many new and well-illustrated titles have appeared and perhaps a small quota from the practice budget for books may be specifically set aside for nursing texts.

Journals and periodicals are a good source of reference material and most practices subscribe to the veterinary titles. What about some specific nursing journals? There are not many available in the UK; however, more are published in the USA where veterinary nurses are known as technicians. Veterinary publications should be available for nurses to see too and, when a member of the vet team spots an appropriate article, the information can be shared.

Books may be considered as rather old-fashioned these days when most individuals are computer-literate, but they are flexible and relatively inexpensive. There are also electronic and visual-learning aids available, such as CDs, DVDs and videos. Some larger conferences and meetings are recorded and audio tapes/CDs etc may be available. Of course, internet access is an added bonus in any library.

Many drug companies produce models and posters for promotional purposes – make the most of these 'freebies' and keep them for all to use. Libraries should be used and sometimes students need a bit of active encouragement to set aside time within the working week to develop personal research skills. Using the library should be part of the practice culture for all the team.

Human resources

This is the most important section in this chapter: nothing happens without people. Whatever the size of the practice, the training of a veterinary nurse is essentially a team effort. Everyone within the working environment should be aware of the role that the practice has chosen to play. The assessor is of course one of the key figures and should be able to organise the student's training and assessment programme.

All training practices need to employ an assessor. As the rules are set by the RCVS the assessor must be qualified to vet or veterinary-nurse level. There are rules also set by the Qualifications and Curriculum Authority (QCA), the government body which guards the educational standards of work-based training (and the whole pre-degree educational system). QCA insists that assessors are trained and qualified to make assessment decisions. It is not just the 'end-point' or outcome that is the training practice's responsibility but the process or how the training takes place. It may seem a little odd that QCA burdens the role of the assessor with the necessity to 'take a qualification' rather than looking to support the actual process of teaching the student.

It is not just the assessor who can offer input to the student. Teaching clinical skills is a rewarding experience and most veterinary personnel enjoy the role of teacher; after all, communicating information and demonstrating techniques to student nurses is not that far removed from teaching clients how to care for their pets. Many vets and nurses have excellent skills in this area. Developing a good clinical-training environment is closely related to the concept of developing good client care. One is an internal part of the business growth and development, the other is external. Unfortunately, the external growth offers very instant and tangible results, whereas internal development is a hidden, rather more long-term, result.

The subject of rotas and time set aside for training and assessment needs to be examined under human resources. This is an important aspect of organisation and duty rotas are often inspected and used as a source of evidence that the veterinary practice is able to confidently support a trainee nurse. Quite clearly, if the assessor is to make accurate decisions concerning the student's competence as a veterinary nurse, they need to work alongside the student for at least two days of the week, if not more. Unfortunately, the best way to provide evidence of the training and assessment process also involves paper records and documentation. Organisational skills are once again a necessary part of successful training.

Sustainability

In conclusion, once the standard for a training practice has been reached, measures need to be taken to ensure these are maintained. Training-practice status is an ongoing process and responsibility. Staff changes can occur quite frequently within a veterinary practice, especially within the nursing team. Having a qualified assessor is essential to maintain training-practice status. It is fast becoming apparent to many training practices that they need more than one assessor within the practice to ensure continuity of training and assessment for their student veterinary nurses. Assessor training is not for everyone but the practice must look for new talent in order to secure the future training of their nursing team.

Student profile 2 Susan

Susan left school and started at the local sixth form studying science-related subjects. After two years it became clear that higher education was not for her. A trainee placement became available at the veterinary practice where she had a Saturday job. Susan applied and became enrolled as a trainee veterinary nurse. She gained her NVQ, qualified as a VN last year and is currently working as Head Nurse. She is looking to enrol for her surgical diploma next year.

4

What is a Veterinary Nurse?

With a heart that never hardens, and a temper that never
tires and a touch that never hurts

A T THIS POINT IT SEEMS appropriate to explore the meaning
of the title of veterinary nurse. How do we know we need one,
let alone undertake the training of a veterinary nurse, if we are
unsure of their function and purpose?

Defining the job

The dictionary definition of nurse is very enlightening:

nurse: *a person trained in the care of the sick; to tend with an eye
to the future, to foster, cherish and cultivate.*

This definition should gladden the heart of any veterinary surgeon
and owner of a small business.

We need to look at a few more definitions to get a clearer all-round
impression of who or what this person can be.

In the USA veterinary nurses are called 'veterinary technicians':

technician: *person skilled in the technique of an art or subject;
person expert in practical application of science; person whose
occupation requires training in specific technical skills and processes.*

There is currently in existence an entry qualification for veterinary nursing – also a qualification standing on its own – that of
animal nursing assistant (previously known as pre–vet nursing).

assistant: *helper, subordinate worker.*

To complete the picture:

veterinary surgeon: *person qualified to examine and treat beasts
medically.*

It is encouraging to see that none of these definitions suggest that the veterinary nurse is a mini-vet. The role of the nurse quite clearly is complementary to that of the veterinary surgeon. Perhaps a definition of our own is needed to add to the dictionary:

> **veterinary nurse**: *a professional person trained in the practical application of the science and art of nursing animals under the care of a veterinary surgeon.*

The skills of the veterinary nurse are acquired to complement and support the work of the veterinary surgeon in a very practical way. As trained individuals they are able to offer a reliable standard of work in areas of client care as well as patient care. Nursing procedures and protocols are important aspects of the job.

A veterinary nurse has a broad base of knowledge with a good basic understanding of the practical side of veterinary science. They are able to carry out a range of skilled activities that assist in both diagnostic and treatment protocols, with the health and welfare of the patient being of primary concern.

Unfortunately, the range of nursing skills routinely used in the workplace can differ widely for individuals. For example, one practice may use the veterinary nurse to support the veterinary team in diagnostic work-ups, such as laboratory tests involving the collection of samples and radiographic procedures, while another practice only uses their nurses for reception, client-care and care of the hospital kennels.

Working as a veterinary nurse can mean something very different from practice to practice. Each veterinary business is a small-business concern that functions as its own little kingdom with internal expectations and protocols, resulting in different levels of nursing practice. However, if the practice employs qualified and trained staff it increasingly makes more economic sense to delegate certain support procedures to a willing and capable nursing team. Standardisation of training practices and the NVQ system has helped to raise the awareness of just how much a veterinary nurse is trained to do.

What are veterinary nurses trained to do?

For full details see the occupational standards for veterinary nursing and the objective syllabus. Here is just a selection of the skills that a certificate-level nurse is able to carry out:

❑ reception and client care
❑ pharmacy and dispensing
❑ patient monitoring
❑ specific nursing care for disease
❑ radiography
❑ anaesthesia–monitoring
❑ fluid therapy
❑ surgical nursing
❑ laboratory work.

It seems a waste (not to mention an expense) if these and other skills are not fully utilised.

The legal aspect

Changes to the Veterinary Surgeons Act 1966 are currently under discussion, with the government working to modernise the laws governing veterinary services. One main area for likely reform of the Act is making provision for non-veterinarians to undertake more procedures currently defined as acts of veterinary surgery. This type of legislation would give veterinary surgeons the power to delegate acts of surgery to anyone holding a recognised qualification.

Veterinary nurses, provided they are listed, are able to carry out certain procedures at the present time. Through the process of listing they are registering as professionals with the RCVS. The training scheme also provides a register of those persons currently undertaking recognised training for the status of veterinary nurse and therefore these individuals are able to carry out basic nursing skills within the remit of the Veterinary Surgeons Act. This new legislation clarifies and tightens up the detail, emphasising and legally recognising – amongst others – the veterinary nurse qualification. This will have some fairly major repercussions for practices which currently employ lay staff who do not hold, or are not working towards, a recognised qualification but are carrying out nursing roles.

Regulation and professional status

Currently, being a listed veterinary nurse carries no true professional status. Veterinary nurses are not regulated. This means, among other things, that there are no requirements for CPD. The 'list' can include the name of a veterinary nurse who has not practiced clinically, for example, for five years or more and has undertaken no CPD. Yet such an individual will still be able to practise, and be employed as a competent nurse, if the retention fee is paid.

If a veterinary nurse acts 'unprofessionally' there are no professional repercussions; their name is still included in the list of veterinary nurses held by the RCVS, providing of course they continue to pay their annual retention fee. I feel that if the veterinary nurse qualification is to be regulated, confidence in the qualification will grow and the veterinary industry will more fully recognise and utilise the skills of the veterinary nurse.

Why practices need to train nurses

Whatever way the debate goes, it is vitally important that veterinary practices appreciate the importance and the advantages of training nurses to a professionally recognised standard. The most effective place to do this is in the clinical environment of the workplace, where useful skills can be taught and practiced to a high level of competence.

In the context of a small business – because that is what most veterinary practices are – the importance of a well-trained and qualified staff has been well documented. In the competitive marketplace, human-resource development plays an important role in the growth and sustainability of a business.

The nursing team is a major part of the resource for a veterinary practice. From the outset, it is important to attract the right sort of individual to join the veterinary team. As with most occupations, veterinary nursing sets its own educational minimum standard as an entry requirement for the qualification. A structure for training is useful as this gives a reliable standard to workplace protocols, both during the process of training and at the final outcome or qualification.

A training structure or ethic in the workplace will also influence the continuing development of the individual, thus developing talents that will benefit the business as a whole. A 'career structure' starts to evolve, which is a motivational factor for some individuals. This is certainly not always easy to achieve and will need good management and organisational skills.

A sense of belonging and teamwork can ensue with loyal and 'bonded' employees who are worth their weight in gold. Veterinary surgeons are always looking to 'bonded' clients as their continuing and reliable source of income: why not apply the concept to human resources and develop a dynamic nursing team?

With recent speculation about a shortage of veterinary nurses, it is important to maintain an ongoing student population in the workplace. If nurses are in such short supply, where will future employees come from? Despite the standardisation of a veterinary nursing qualification, 'home grown' nurses are the best. They will already have the practice ethic and specific practice protocols well rehearsed, as well as the RCVS professional stamp of approval.

Training a veterinary nurse does take time and effort but the rewards can be many and far-reaching.

A Veterinary Nurse is   Very Naughty
Very Nice
Very Necessary.

From bio-security to client care every practice needs veterinary nurses. To be of practical use, they need to be practically tutored and trained in the workplace: it is really not that difficult.

Assessor profile 2 Simon

Simon is a practice principal and employs only two members of staff. He holds his assessor certificate and has just managed to support his two students through their NVQ in veterinary nursing. It was a struggle and luckily both his students were mature and very motivated. They had to visit a neighboring practice to gain the necessary range of experience for the radiography and laboratory module.

Simon had decided that he would relinquish his training-practice status, particularly as both his nurses are now qualified. However, he has recently received a request from a student following the degree route for veterinary nursing. He is considering acting as a host practice for this student and retaining his TP status, particularly as an extra pair of hands during the summer could be useful.

5

The Team

Success comes in cans – not can'ts

FANTASTIC, YOU ARE STILL READING and still enthusiastic about wanting to train veterinary nurses. In previous chapters we have discussed the physical resources of the practice and now we need to look at the members of the team who will provide the human resource.

The players

Teamwork in the workplace is so important and plays a very important part in the success of any business. Therefore it will be of no surprise that the whole team in the veterinary workplace should play a vital role in the success of a training practice. The main 'players' are of course the assessor and the student, but the other staff members are a valuable resource for them.

In studying the content of the NVQ veterinary nursing syllabus and portfolio work, one quickly appreciates the breadth of skills and knowledge that the student needs to acquire. Who better to impart these skills than the 'experts' in their field? All the practice members need to understand what is involved in training a student veterinary nurse and to be encouraged to participate. In particular, they all need to be familiar with the units of competence that have to be achieved by each student before they can claim their veterinary nurse status.

Reception duty features quite heavily in Level 2 and who better to teach some of the finer points of customer care than your

experienced reception-
ists? Laboratory skills
feature in Level 3
– every practice has
a white-coated 'bof-
fin' in the lab who
does amazing
things with the
microscope. The
practice manager
is often
steeped in
the mysteries of
health and safety
and can assist with
the finer points for
those particular portfolio log
sheets.

Of course, it is the assessor who has to assess and judge competency against the standards, but that does not stop others assisting
with the input before the final 'test'. Many will find that they enjoy
having a student to nurture and that it will help to keep their theory
and practice alive and kicking – possibly refreshing parts that have
long since faded into obscurity.

This all sounds very jolly, but its success will depend upon the
organisational and communication skills of the assessor. Do not
for one moment think that successful training and assessment is
confined to the resources of large highly efficient hospital-type
veterinary teams. In fact, internal communication needs to be
working at a high level and that can sometimes be quite a challenge
within a large bustling environment. It can be that smaller and
more tight-knit practices with only a few staff members can manage communication easily and more effectively, where the student
and assessor can benefit from a more individual training experience.
Small but perfectly formed practice teams can be just as successful
and in some cases are even better.

Star players
The assessor

As part of the practice management strategy, it is a good idea to outline the role of assessor with a specific job description giving detail of duties and responsibilities. The job description needs to be quite clear about how much time is to be allocated to the assessor if the RCVS requirements are to be met and effective training to take place.

Very often head nurses are left to undertake the role of assessor with little thought given to the extra workload that this will involve. From experience, the head nurse is a very busy member of the team dealing with staff rotas, drug ordering and repair of equipment, not to mention nursing duties and management meetings that need to be attended – there are just not enough hours in the day.

Likewise practice principals, with the best will in the world, do not have the time – or patience – to devote the necessary hours to the training and assessment of a student veterinary nurse. There are of course exceptions, but they are very few and far between and generally to be found within the smaller practice setup.

Figure 5   **Wanted – Assessor**

Must have:
- [ ] good organisational skills
- [ ] ability to communicate
- [ ] desire to train future members of our nursing team
- [ ] flexibility and innovative approach
- [ ] patience
- [ ] knowledge of current nursing practice.

If the practice supports a number of veterinary surgeons with a good team of qualified nursing staff, the role of the assessor can be successfully used to create an internal 'career structure'. Many practices successfully train up a good team of qualified nurses and then feel frustrated when they leave to discover pastures new. Your newly qualified fully-fledged veterinary nurses will naturally look to move to a workplace that will offer more responsibility and a more senior position. These 'home grown' nurses are a valuable asset to the veterinary business and efforts need to be made to keep them on board.

It is unfortunate that the role of head nurse is often held by one individual for a number of years and seen as the only role with responsibility in the nursing team. Wise practices have looked at developing roles in surgery and preventative health care in an attempt to retain their qualified nurses. The demands of the NVQ assessment system have created an important new role, offering individuals a chance to use their nursing knowledge and experience while developing a whole new range of skills associated with assessing and training. Wise management teams should look closely at this emerging role – it may be of some interest.

Veterinary surgeons must not be discounted from this role, as there are some excellent vet assessors in many training practices. Again, they need this extra role to be recognised as a scheduled part of their duty rota and to have the full support of the practice principal. From a business perspective it may be very hard to justify the use of a veterinary surgeon's time to this end. Vets, possibly, have a harder task assessing veterinary nurses; although the two professions complement each other, they are in fact quite different jobs, with somewhat different levels of understanding. Nurses are not mini-vets and need to acquire a different set of work-based skills to complement the higher skill level of practising veterinary medicine.

In conclusion, the best person for the role of assessor is the qualified veterinary nurse. They will have the desire and motivation to
pass on their skills and knowledge and ensure a high standard of
nursing care is maintained within the veterinary practice. If you are
lucky, these star players are already present within the nursing team.
Of course, the RCVS rules and regulations need to be followed and
it is advisable for the assessor to have at least one year's practical
experience as a qualified nurse before undertaking the role of the
assessor. Often, however, it is the recently qualified professional
who is bursting to share new-found knowledge and confidence.

The student

It seems that there is no shortage of individuals wishing to 'work
with animals'. The majority of practices receive at least two letters
a week from hopefuls. It would be easy to presume that with all
this interest in working in the veterinary industry there would not
be any difficulty in finding the right person for the role of student
within the team. However, it often transpires that many applicants
are quite inappropriate, if not from the lack of entry requirements,
then from the point of view of their expectations. Perhaps the latest
television documentaries have had some influence here?

It is important to select your prospective student with care, as
each practice should with any new employee, ensuring that they
understand the training process and their own roles and responsibilities. Again, the purposes of the job description and person
specification come to mind.

Everyone needs to be aware of what is expected of them. Your
veterinary nurse student will have two roles – an employee in the
workplace and a trainee veterinary nurse. Likewise, the employer
has two roles to play – the employer and the workplace trainer.
Admittedly, the college course plays a supporting role here, but
the workplace skills and assessments are the responsibility of the
employer. It is so important to get these roles and responsibilities
defined and understood at the start of the 'apprentice' training
period. Students particularly need to understand these roles and
adopt the right attitude within the workplace.

The HE student

Veterinary nursing is a very practical skill and the workplace or shop floor is the ideal place to learn. A few students may be following a degree or HE course that involves veterinary nurse training as part of the final qualification. These students require clinical placements in a training practive in order to collect evidence to meet the occupational standards for veterinary nursing laid down by the RCVS. As a general rule these students are regarded as 'extras' to the nursing team and many do not require payment.

It must be remembered that they are in the workplace to be trained and that will involve the same type of input, time and assessment opportunities that a more traditional apprentice-NVQ student requires. This type of HE student is there to actively learn and practise the art and skills of veterinary nursing, albeit in a more intense time frame. It is essential that the veterinary team and also the student understand their roles within this HE framework for the Veterinary Nursing Certificate.

Student profile 3   David

David wanted to study animal science at university. He started a four-year degree course that included an NVQ in veterinary nursing. He managed to find a work placement in a large veterinary hospital which enabled him to meet the requirements for the NVQ.

Although he enjoyed the work very much he realised that, once he had his degree, he would prefer to work as a representative for a drug company. He has achieved his VN qualification but he has one year left on his degree course and he is already looking for opportunities in the commercial field.

Student profile 4   Jane

Jane attended a career evening during her years at sixth form and decided that she would like to follow a degree course that included veterinary nursing. It was during her first year, whilst on work placement, that she discovered that she could obtain her VN qualification via a work-based route.

She really enjoyed her work placement and realised she had a very practical nature. Her host practice was losing one of their nurses and Jane decided to take the opportunity to change to a work-based NVQ course. She was employed by the training practice and has just completed her Level 2 NVQ and is starting on her Level 3 coursework later this year. Jane has settled well to a day-release college course and, unlike her friends who stayed on at university, she is now earning a wage rather than increasing her student debt.

6

How the Qualification Works

The greatest failure is the failure to try

WITH ALL THE OFFICIAL PAPERWORK and documentation that goes with work based training it is easy to lose sight of the intended goal – the reliable assessment of a trainee veterinary nurse, and of the ultimate goal – a professionally competent individual who will be an asset to the veterinary team and business. It is important to hang on to that ultimate goal for the assessor, student and the practice.

At this point we will look at the collection of evidence and the assessment process before moving on to pointers on how to support training and assessment in the workplace with an organised system.

What is assessing all about?
Simply put, assessors measure an individual's competence against a set of occupational standards established by the relevant professional body. So for the VN qualification, the assessors are using the documented standards for veterinary nursing to ensure that each student is well-practised, skilled and safe to carry out nursing procedures.

It is so important that everyone understands this – especially the students! They are provided with a copy of the standards with their portfolio and they need to read them. Likewise, assessors need to read and acquaint themselves with the standards and the scope (or range, as it used to be called) of experience that the student must undergo. The other piece of essential reading is the portfolio itself, along with the front prefaces and any annexes. Each training practice should have their own copy of these printed documents.

They are available for download from the RCVS website or by post from the veterinary nursing department (see Useful Addresses at the end of this book). There are a few other publications on the veterinary market with hints and tips on how to complete log sheets but you could save your time and money and read the 'latest' version: it is the best and most detailed. Taking a little more time to read these documents at an early stage will pay dividends in the future.

Warning 1

You will not be able to survive without a full copy of the portfolio and standards

---

The function and role of the portfolio

The portfolio has been developed by the RCVS as the vehicle to be used by the student and the assessor to offer evidence of the trainee's competence within their role as a veterinary nurse. This is not the page or chapter in which to discuss the merits or shortcomings of this system. Instead we need to look at how to use the portfolio to our best advantage without creating too many problems for ourselves or our students.

The portfolio is used to provide evidence of a level of nursing care that meets the standards set by the awarding body – the RCVS. It needs to meet the full range or scope of experience required for veterinary nursing ensuring that each successful student has truly met the standard.

The modules

The portfolio is divided up into modules, each containing a series of log sheets that need to be completed as evidence of the student's ability in the workplace. These log sheets are for collection of evidence that is dynamic and, if completed as instructed (see Portfolio pointers later in this chapter), they should cover the units and elements of the occupational standards.

Unfortunately, during the last revision of the portfolio the numbering of the modules and the units were not streamlined well and it can be confusing to try matching modules to the units. Again, if you have read your portfolio you will be aware of the comprehensive guidance notes that exist at the start of every module and full reference is made to the relevant units.

The number of log sheets has been extensively criticized, but their number is partly dictated by the range of evidence that is required by each unit. A full range of species and case types needs to be included within the modules. As experience grows with portfolio-building it becomes apparent that many valid 'short cuts' can be taken. If all the units and elements can be covered on fewer log sheets then so much the better.

As long as the assessor keeps a record of what exactly has been covered from the standards much repetition can be avoided. A simple checklist or indeed a copy of the standards with a tick beside each element or performance criteria would suffice. Reference in the margin of the log sheet can be made to the unit or element that has been checked. If the scope or range has not been fully met then questions can be used and a record of these can also be made in the margin.

Each element of the standards contains a brief outline of the types of questions that can be used by the assessor. It must be remembered that evidence for one unit might meet the requirements for another unit, thus cross-referencing will reduce the workload.

It is important that the student veterinary nurse loses the 'school project' approach and moves towards the more adult techniques of evidence-collecting. So many nursing students spend hours and hours on the aesthetic aspects of their portfolio rather than concentrating on how to make the most use of evidence available to them. Some assessors are equally at fault here, often demanding over-detailed log sheets and requiring that every log sheet be word-processed. It is perfectly acceptable for the logs to be completed in bullet points as, after all, they are a brief diary of events and a record of the student's capabilities.

Assessors need to support their students and guide them towards the collection of relevant work-based evidence as well as giving instruction on the art and skill of cross-referencing!

Collecting appropriate and valid work-based evidence

Making sure work-based evidence is valid and appropriate is the point when assessors have to look to their assessor training, where different types of valid evidence were discussed. Items such as work-product evidence, witness statements, direct observations, photographs and sometimes video and oral tape evidence are all valid.

Monitoring charts

For veterinary nursing the biggest source of 'natural' evidence presents itself in the form of patient-monitoring charts. A word of caution here – be very aware of the detail that is presented on these charts. I have found that many practices, although they keep charts, do not complete them fully or skimp on the detail. It may be necessary to look critically at the detail on monitoring charts and perhaps adapt the information collected to meet the evidence requirements of the standards.

For example, it is amazing how many hospital charts in routine use do not carry regular recording of parameters such as temperature, pulse and respiration. The boxes are there but no values appear to be recorded. Quite clearly a hospital chart would be excellent evidence of nursing care given to support a patient; however, its validity and relevance would be called into question if the detail was missing.

Perhaps this is a good time for practices to look at their in-house patient care and tighten up the monitoring process. If a good level of care is routinely practised, collection of valid and relevant evidence will be easy for veterinary nursing students. Assessors will have an easy and guaranteed valid source of evidence that can be used across various modules. It is worth spending time 'upgrading' the practice charts – hospital in-patients, intensive care, fluid monitoring, anaesthetic monitoring and post-anaesthetic recovery charts, to suggest a few.

Witness statements

These are also very useful, but need to be used correctly. It is perfectly possible for the student to have carried out some nursing routine with colleagues who do not hold the assessor qualification. At this time a statement of actions and observations of the process can be formally presented in writing and included with the written log sheet. The assessor is still required to sign the log sheet, as assessed, and they use the witness statement to support the evidence. Witness statements should not form the bulk of the evidence within each module.

Photographs

These are a good form of evidence, especially if a digital camera is available, but it is still very much a question of being in the right place at the right time.

Direct observations

Collecting evidence directly becomes easier with time and experience. Remember to plan this properly to get maximum benefit from the task and always link this with the collection of a supporting log sheet to save time.

Systems and control

It cannot be emphasised too often that each working veterinary practice is different with different organisational protocols. This very point underlines the need for a flexible training and assessment system that can succeed in every workplace. Generally, this was the aim and the ideology behind the NVQ system. The RCVS sets the basic minimum requirements for human and physical resources in the training practices. Within this infrastructure the assessment process can be customised to suit the individual practice, providing the standards are met. This is great news, and with a little effort and imagination, veterinary nurse training is possible in almost every practice.

Communication

One of the biggest hurdles to overcome is that of communication. In general, communication is the key to any successful venture and it is not easy. There are lots of publications covering this topic and these make valuable reading. If the practice has the opportunity to attend a workshop or seminar dealing with communication, do go. It is important that the whole practice attends, from the boss to the cleaner.

Within the practice, communicating the practice's role as a TP is vital: everyone who works in a training environment must be aware of the processes involved in training a student veterinary nurse. They may not play an active role in training but they need to understand the involvement and responsibilities of those who do. In a busy working environment people can become impatient when temporary changes are made to their working schedule, if they do not understand the need to carry out assessments etc. With good planning and communication any changes can be brief and cause minimum disruption to the working schedule.

Figure 6	Example of planning flexibly to include assessment

❏ An extension of ten minutes to the morning coffee break, to allow a direct assessment to be carried out on a Level 2 student, preparing and setting up a drip to complete Unit 2 of the vn Standards.

❏ The student arriving ten minutes before the start of the shift for assessment in giving routine medication to a hospitalised patient.

❏ A change of duty from the kennels to reception for a short period to enable assessor to complete assessment of skills in client care.

So the list could go on. Of course, the above changes will involve the assessor as well as the student. This can be a problem if the assessor is the veterinary surgeon; however, nothing is impossible. Negotiation and planning will be skills that are required here, but that should not be too problematic as long as the whole practice is committed and understands the need for training.

Meetings

Everyone hates meetings, probably because they feel that they are a waste of time and invariably nothing gets done. It can be different. Meetings about training need to be held at regular intervals. How often and how long will be determined by the individual practices. In the large practice, with maybe two assessors and three students, meetings will need to be held more frequently and will probably take a little longer. In the smaller, more compact practice, the assessor and student work daily together and progress and planning meetings are easier to set up.

A clear agenda for each meeting will help to keep the discussion concise and help with finishing on time. The art of good meetings requires some organisation and experience, but once they have developed a pattern and become part of practice life, things get easier and their value becomes apparent. These meetings should deal with planning and the progress of your students' assessment and training.

Figure 7	Starting to meet as you mean to go on

❏ So you are starting off with a new NVQ student (or maybe two) – begin as you mean to go on.

❏ Plan a set time within your working week that is specifically for 'training and portfolio work'. You book appointment times for clients – why not do the same for training? You look after your clients with practised skill – why not look after the nursing team with the same practised skill?

❏ OK, so weekly is difficult – how about once every two weeks?

❏ Organisation – that's what is needed. Once started, keep to a regular pattern and it will soon become part of practice life. Look long term at this; it is going to take two years at least to complete the training for one student and by then it will be time to enrol the next.

Agendas

Once you have set the appointment times over the next few months, perhaps even for the next few years, what are you going to do in the allotted time with your student? This part is important, as it needs to be concise.

Long-term planning is a good place to start. Get a feel for the portfolio as a whole and look at the number of logs that need to be completed and the scope and range of evidence that is required. Think about how and when you will be able to carry out formal assessments on your student. Find out what is being taught at college and link the modules with the knowledge input.

Communicate with your student. This is most important because it is, after all, their qualification and they need to take responsibility for their own work. Many students take a while to understand this principle and sometimes I think it is because the assessor becomes very much the controlling force. Remember this is not your portfolio. Your role is to guide and assess the competency of your student to a national standard.

Continuing on the subject of roles, it has been my experience that a number of trainee veterinary nurses forget that they are employees in the first instance and students in the second. It is important that the right attitude is adopted at the outset by both the student and the assessor to avoid any unnecessary conflicts of interest.

Figure 8	A basic sample agenda

1   Progress since last meeting
   ➪ Keep tracking sheet up to date, check and assess log sheets presented.

2   Plan the next move
   ➪ Look at what evidence is still outstanding: log sheets or direct assessments.
   ➪ Discuss ideas for case types and any supporting evidence that is relevant such as detailed hospital charts etc.
   ➪ Think about how cases may be cross-referenced to fulfill the evidence requirements for another module.
   ➪ Are there any appropriate members of the team who could act as witnesses or evidence-gatherers?

3   Any problems or issues that need to be resolved?

Keep a record or diary of these meetings as this is part of the assessment process and the training practice's evidence that the student is being supported.

Of course, if there is more than one assessor the assessor team will need to meet at frequent intervals to plan the division of responsibility for each of the students in the practice and discuss the progress of individuals.

Most practices have a regular system of meetings within the practice organisation and it is always beneficial if such meetings carry 'training' as an item on the agenda. Then everyone can be kept informed in outline about the progress of the students. Lines of communication need to be kept open.

Record-keeping and paperwork

On the face of it, the system of work-based training appears to have created mountains of paperwork. In fact, this is because we – the creators of the paper – need to be more organised and selective in our work.

The records that are needed are quite simple and, if kept in a loose-leaf folder in one specific place, there should be no problems. There are two sets of papers for each student:

❑ the first is the student's own portfolio of evidence

❑ the second is the training practice's evidence of the training and assessment of the student.

At this point we will assume that the student has taken responsibility for their own paperwork and we will look at what the training practice and the assessor need to keep.

Figure 9   Training practice's evidence of the training

1 Training practice number as granted by the VNAC
2 Details and contact for internal verifier through VNAC
3 Details of assessor's qualifications and CPD
4 Details of the student's enrolment date and number with the awarding body
5 Copy of the student's record of employment
6 Details of the college course attended by the student and any reports received
7 Tracking sheet for portfolio logs
8 Tracking sheet of direct assessments carried out to cover the units/ elements
9 Direct assessments – planning, task and feedback sheet for each
10 Record of meetings and training sessions with student held in practice
11 Copy of module summary sheets when each module and the relevant units have been completed.

Once this information has been collected any further documents can be added as they are produced. It is just a question of getting organised, developing a system and becoming the controller of the paper.

Communication tips

Notice boards

These can be in staff rooms or in the central work area of the practice, e.g. the preparation area. Tracking sheets can be kept accessible to ensure that the whole team is aware of their students' progress. The notice board can also be used to request case types that are needed to complete modules or ranges of evidence. This gives other members of the veterinary team the opportunity to act as 'evidence gatherers' or witnesses to the students' experience and nursing skills when maybe the assessor is not present, or on another shift. You do not want to miss that 'naturally occurring' evidence.

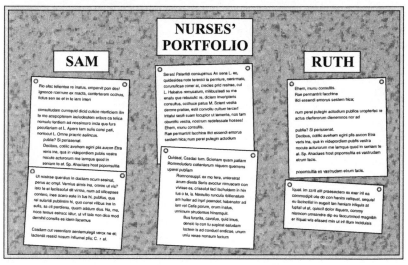

Use of internal email

Basically, this involves using an electronic notice board. As with any notice board keep neat and tidy and constantly update it – a dynamic tool.

Practice meetings

❑ Always include an item marked 'training' on the agenda to keep the whole practice informed of plans and progress.

❑ Regular meetings of the assessor team, again for planning and progress.

❑ Regular meetings with students.

Remember that as a training practice you have undertaken to provide a minimum of three hours' training support a week.

External communication

As a training practice you are not acting in isolation – you are part of a larger group or VNAC, which is there to help. An internal verifier will be available for support and advice regarding training and assessment. Every assessor should have the support of an internal verifier, who they can easily contact for advice no matter how trivial it may be. As an internal verifier, I enjoy hearing from my assessors and sometimes it is great just to know that they are still alive and kicking. Try to attend the regular meetings that are held by the

VNACs for their training practices.

I know it is always a great effort to attend these external meetings, adding constraints on the working day, but besides being a requirement of training practice status they are a great opportunity.

❑ Meet and share problems with other assessors.

    ➭ How do you deal with the unwilling student?

    ➭ How to deal with all the paperwork?

❑ Keep up to date with any changes that have occurred within the NVQ system.

    ➭ Changes can be made by QCA, who influence the RCVS, and on decisions concerning levels and type of evidence that is necessary for the NVQ in veterinary nursing.

❑ These meetings also help to standardise the competency levels expected for veterinary nursing.

    ➭ We all get a little rusty, even with regular CPD. It is a little like driving the car – we all develop our own personal short cuts that might not precisely meet national standards.

The standards for veterinary nursing explain the evidence our students need to present, but there are no details of technique or 'how to do it'. That is where our own professional expertise comes into play and it is for this reason that assessors for veterinary nursing must be appropriately qualified. Continuing professional development is an important part of the professional ethic and it plays an important supportive role for those who are acting as assessors.

For example, what exactly is the correct method of putting on a pair of sterile gloves? How do you focus the microscope for that blood smear? Keep up to date with current nursing practice – to be honest it does not change drastically. Attending regular assessor meetings provides the ideal opportunities to revise the finer key points and develop good working practices.

Veterinary nursing students currently still have to pass a practical examination at Level 3 before they are able to claim listed status and good practical training in the workplace will go a long way towards their individual levels of success.

Portfolio pointers

The following tips may prove useful for assessors and students when approaching their nursing portfolios for the first time.

The aim and purpose of the portfolio is to provide a body of work that offers reliable evidence of the student's actions and experiences in the workplace during the prescribed training period. The modules and log sheets have been designed in such a way that, if completed correctly, they meet the full range/scope of experience required to reach the occupational standards. More detailed information on the individual log sheets can be found in the pages marked 'Guidance notes for student and assessor' in the RCVS Veterinary Nursing Portfolio.

Figure 10   **Portfolio hints and tips**

❏ Keep 'Guidance Notes' handy for easy reference – they provide the answers to most problems.
❏ Make sure your student reads and understands what is required.
❏ Remember to collect any additional evidence requested.
❏ Remember to refer to the occupational standards for the finer detail.

Cross-referencing cases will help reduce the workload for both students and assessors and also provide a more holistic approach to the portfolio. It is possible, especially at Level 3, to use the nursing actions carried out for one patient to cover a whole range of log sheets, therefore providing evidence for more than one unit.

For example, it may be possible to use a patient with a 'pyometra' to cover Laboratory, Fluid Therapy, Anaesthesia and Surgical Nursing logs. Be sure to clearly reference the evidence to the relevant log sheets. Evidence on the log sheets needs to be clear and concise so that when internal verification is carried out nothing will be missed.

Information collected to be used to demonstrate the underpinning knowledge and understanding of any cases used for the portfolio log sheets should be acknowledged in the 'comments' section. For example, a reference/text book, a CD or the internet may have been used to check the nursing care of some exotic breed of reptile. It is perfectly acceptable to acknowledge help and assistance given by experienced members of staff, such as vets and nurses, who hold higher qualifications.

Different types of supporting evidence may be used within the modules alongside the log sheets. Remember that the evidence must be valid. For example, a printed brochure provided by a drug company giving information on a prescription diet is not appropriate. What is required are items such as hospital sheets, notes made when monitoring a trauma patient or one requiring some intensive care and anaesthetic charts. It is important to understand that any additional or supporting evidence must be as a result of the student's own efforts. The assessor must sign and date these extra documents to authenticate their originality.

Figure 11   **Valid supporting work-based product evidence**

❏ Hospital/monitoring charts
   Perhaps highlight the nursing care specifically carried out by one person.
❏ Consent forms
   Ensure that confidentiality is carefully observed.
❏ Dispensing labels
   Ensure that confidentiality is maintained.
❏ Anaesthetic charts
❏ Laboratory results sheets
❏ Drug/stock orders
❏ Witness statements
   Remember to collect any signatures on the authentication sheet.
❏ Photographs
❏ Information leaflets specifically produced by the student for practice use
❏ Written reports – as requested in Level 3.

Appendices will prove useful for many of the modules. For example, in Level 2 the Basic Nursing module contains logs that evidence the care of hospitalised patients. The section that deals with cleaning animal accommodation will probably be the same for most of the logs. Creating a correctly detailed appendix that outlines the student's actions within the practice protocol and precautions taken with regard to health and safety will save a lot of time and effort. The assessor needs to be aware that some further detail regarding cleaning and disinfection may be necessary on logs dealing with exotic or infectious patients to meet the range/scope of experience evidenced in the logs.

Each appendix should be produced by the student for the first log sheet that it supports. The assessor will need to see the appendix before assessing the written log sheet evidence. It is not valid practice for the student to complete the appendix at the end of the module. Each appendix should carry the assessor's signature and the date of the first log sheet to which it pertains.

Figure 12 **Suggested Level 2 appendices**

❑ Prepare and assist with procedures (Module 4)
- ➭ preparation of the clinical environment
- ➭ disposal of waste/sharps etc
- ➭ health and safety.

❑ Basic nursing (Module 5)
- ➭ cleaning and disinfectant protocol
- ➭ type of accommodation used, perhaps to include a plan of kennel area showing sizes and location
- ➭ types of bedding used.

Figure 13 **Suggested Level 3 appendices**

❑ Surgical nursing (Module 9)
- ➭ list of instruments in a basic surgical kit
- ➭ skin preparation routine
- ➭ drapes commonly used
- ➭ preparation of the surgical team
- ➭ routine post-operative nursing.

❑ Anaesthesia (Module 10)
- ➭ routine preparation of anaesthetic equipment
- ➭ routine cleaning and care of equipment

Assessor profile 3   Fiona

Last year, veterinary nurse Fiona was literally 'tearing her hair out' with her Level 2 trainee. Alice had been employed by the practice for six months and enrolled on the RCVS scheme. Alice was attending a block-release course and had successfully completed the first block. Her report was good and the end-of-session exam results were promising. However, at work Alice lacked motivation and did not seem to understand the need to collect work-based evidence for her portfolio.

Fiona had agreed a good action plan with Alice and regular tutorials were held. Fiona became very concerned with lack of progress and contacted her internal verifier at the VNAC. Fiona was advised to continue to keep written documentation of tutorials and lack of progress made with the student. A month later an internal verification visit was arranged with the assessor, student and practice manager.

The internal verifier found that despite regular tutorials and plenty of opportunity to collect evidence, the student had made no real progress. The practice manager was also becoming concerned at the demotivating effect the student was having on the rest of the team. During the interview it became apparent that Alice was not enjoying her work in practice and was considering leaving veterinary nursing.

It was decided that the practice would delay her VN training and attendance at college for six months. Alice decided to leave the practice and she is now studying for A levels at the local college. The practice, and in particular Fiona, were quite skeptical about training another student through the NVQ route. However due to lack of qualified nurses they found they had to employ another trainee. Fiona cannot believe how easy it is working and training a motivated and eager student. She is really enjoying her role as assessor and she is looking to expanding her skills further by taking a basic teaching course at night school.

7

The Role of the Veterinary Nursing Approved Centre

Growth begins when we start to accept our own
weakness

THE VETERINARY NURSING APPROVED CENTRE provides
an umbrella of support to a group of training practices. The
VNAC's primary role is to ensure that the assessment decisions made
by individual assessors about the competence of their student nurses are standardised. This is done through the internal verification
process. Despite their title, internal verifiers ensure quality control
from outside the practice. In a larger organization – a company, NHS
hospital or college – they would be 'internal' to the training function; in veterinary practices, as with other small businesses, they are
actually 'external'.

Internal verification
Internal verifiers (IVs) are well-qualified veterinary professionals
who also hold a qualification for internal verification. They are
required to visit each training practice to monitor the quality of
work-based training the individual student is receiving. They are
able to offer support and advice to assessors and to help with the
organisation of all the paperwork. The internal verifier may even
have a few ideas for reducing that mountain of paper.

The visits
The internal verifier works under the watchful eye of the RCVS and

QCA to 'check out' the progress of each student and the work of the assessor. To monitor these activities they have to visit the training practice at regular intervals to directly observe the work-based training and assessments.

The internal verifier needs to be certain that each student's portfolio of evidence is a true representation of nursing skills achieved. QCA demands authentic, reliable and current evidence and someone has to check to make sure that it is not all being made up. Needless to say, the visits by the internal verifier are not overly popular, as not many of us enjoy being inspected.

It is far better to look upon these visits as a chance for support and advice. As a relationship is built up between the assessor and the internal verifier everything becomes much more enjoyable. Of course some of the points raised by the internal verifier may not be to the liking of the training practice. But if the practice wishes to be involved with training, it may have to make certain changes to practice protocols. If changes have to be made, action plans are usually drawn up and a further visit will be required to establish compliance. Usually, problems are easily resolved.

Examples of IVs in action

❏ The practice may not routinely use anaesthetic charts for monitoring patients. If they do not, students have difficulty in collecting the necessary evidence for the anaesthesia module. By introducing the regular use of such charts, all the personnel involved with monitoring patients (and not only the students) will become proficient in this skill, and collection of the necessary evidence will be very simple.

❏ Although the practice has a separate preparation area and a separate theatre, the current theatre protocol 'cuts corners' and patients are anaesthetised and clipped up in the theatre in an attempt to save time, rather than following a more appropriate aseptic protocol by using the prep area.

We all learn to take short cuts in our working life but things need to be done 'properly' in the training environment.

The process of checking, or verification, unfortunately has to generate its own evidence – a few more bits of paper. One of the most useful functions of the internal verifier is to help organise and shuffle all these pieces of paper. It is quite simple really – collect all the generated paperwork and keep it in a file that is available at any time for inspection by any official person that wishes to read it.

The paperwork

These are your records and proof of the fantastic job you and your practice are doing in the training of your student veterinary nurse. What should be kept?

❑ Evidence of assessor qualifications.
❑ Details of student enrolment on the RCVS training scheme, including date etc.
❑ Tracking sheet of progress made with the portfolio logs and evidence collected towards the individual units
❑ Copy of the student's employment record along with details of time off for sickness and holidays.
   This item may be filed with whoever is in charge of human resources at the practice – generally the practice manager. It needs to be kept up to date as this is an important document. It records the time served as a trainee in practice; for a veterinary nurse the apprenticeship period is 94 weeks. (The employment record is to be found in the front pages of the portfolio.)
❑ Record of tutorials and teaching sessions that the student has received.
   It is important to have regular meetings between the assessor and student to update records and discuss progress with the collection of portfolio evidence. A simple diary format is all that is needed and this can be the responsibility of the student as much as that of the assessor. If outside meetings or even congresses are attended these should be recorded. CPD is applicable to qualified professionals and students alike. Some practices have a good internal system for CPD with regular training sessions held within the practice; once again all of this is evidence and counts towards the student's training experience.

❏ Paperwork that relates to direct observations of tasks set for the student and used by the assessor to ensure that they have been assessed as competent in all the units of the standards. This usually consists of a task sheet that relates directly to the standards, a set of oral questions and answers and, of course, some type of feedback and report.

❏ Module summary sheets
On completion of the modules for the portfolio, the assessor has to complete a final report – currently known as the 'module summary sheet'. A copy of this needs to be kept as evidence of the assessment process. The training practice does not need to keep a copy of the whole portfolio.

❏ Reports that have been received from the internal verifier.

Portfolio reviews

A good way of checking that training and assessment is taking place to the national standard is to look at what is produced, i.e. the portfolio. The student's portfolio contains evidence of their experiences and skill levels. The log sheets also reflect the assessment process.

The portfolio is reviewed during what is referred to as the 'building stage' and also again at the end point. The mid-point review is the most productive one and at this stage any problems can be picked up. From a report that is generated by the internal verifier, the assessor can further advise and guide the student with the collection of relevant evidence to complete the portfolio to the national standard. In effect the portfolio cannot 'fail'. If it does not reach the required standard the student is requested to submit the missing items of evidence before the final verification report is generated.

Standardisation meetings

As part of its support for assessors, the VNAC has to develop its team of assessors and pay close attention to the principle of quality control. Every assessor is working with the same set of occupational standards that have been set by the awarding body – the RCVS. As always with anything of a highly practical nature the problem is the level of interpretation of the written word. It is important that

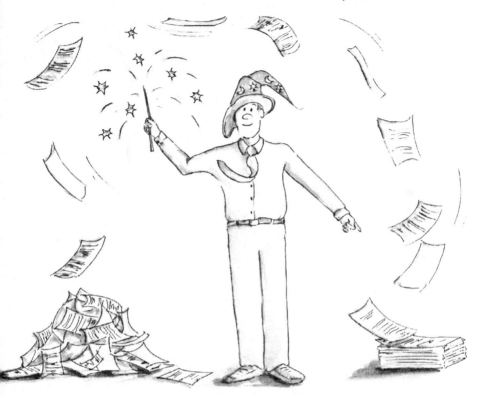

assessors are familiar with the content of the standards. They must be able to identify key nursing skills in which the student needs to be competent in order to function as a veterinary nurse.

These meetings play a part in raising awareness and standardising assessment decisions. Role-plays often form a part of the timetable, with essential skills being demonstrated and assessed, set up rather like the practical examination task. Another useful way of standard-ising log sheets is to carry out a critique of a set of log sheets that have been assessed by an anonymous assessor. It is very helpful to see 'how others do it'. The workshop sessions often generate a lot of interesting detail and they provide a good opportunity for assessors to share individual problems and concerns.

Who are the vnacs?

Each veterinary practice that wishes to train student nurses must seek out a VNAC to provide the necessary service of internal verification. The choice of VNAC may be influenced by a number of factors, not least its geographical location. As internal verification visits have to be made at reasonably frequent intervals, with more visits if there are problems, mileage expenses have to be built into the fee for this service. There has to be a charge to meet the cost of this service, although fees are generally quite reasonable.

Each VNAC is inspected and approved by the RCVS working to QCA's regulations for external verification. Essentially, all the services they provide have to be standard and each establishment is visited and inspected on a regular basis – quality control all over again.

❑ VNACs may be linked to a college or course provider for veterinary nurses. This can have the advantage that the tutors may also be the IVs, providing the opportunity for greater continuity of training and communication with assessors.

❑ A group or consortium of practices could be formed to organise their own internal verification and share in the costs this process inevitably incurs. (Very often professional jealousy prevents this being possible or as successful as it might be.)

❑ A very large practice for example – a veterinary hospital – may be able to support more than one student, a whole team of assessors and one designated internal verifier. With such a large staff it may be possible to find all the necessary 'cast' members.

❑ There are a number of small private training companies that provide VNAC services.

A full current list of VNACs is available from the RCVS Veterinary Nursing web site; a list at the time of writing can be found in Appendix 2.

External verification

This is the final process in the chain of quality control and validation of the process of work-based training as an integral part of the Veterinary Nursing Certificate. A team of external verifiers work on behalf of the RCVS to ensure that the whole system works to the standards set by the QCA and the relevant interested awarding bodies and government education departments.

The external verifiers are all well-qualified veterinary profession-als with an interest in education and training. They need to find evidence of a standardised assessment process so they look hard at the VNACs and the internal verification process. They gather evidence from paperwork and records and by directly observing the whole nurse-training programme in action, and of course they study completed portfolios. The external verifiers also hold their own type of standardisation meetings for internal verifiers to ensure that everyone is working to the national standard. Standards of work-based training are monitored through the process as well as the outcome.

Student profile 5   Angela

Angela was employed as a trainee in a very busy training practice. Angela soon found that she was unable to keep up with the busy pace of the practice and fell behind with her portfolio logs. She was able to speak to her tutors at college and her problems were highlighted to the VNAC. The internal verifier approached the assessor within the training practice and discussed Angela's problems. It was found that the TP was finding it difficult to support Angela fully due to lack of time.

Various solutions were discussed and it was agreed that the nurses' rota would include a specified time for student and assessor to work in the practice library undisturbed. This was set at an hour a week. It was difficult at first but, once the whole practice understood the type of support their student needed, things became a lot easier. Other members of staff became interested in supporting Angela with her study and now the assessor spends roughly half the allocated time with the student dealing with log sheets and assessments. The rest of the study time is organised around volunteer members of staff who are eager to impart their knowledge.

8

Common Problems and Concerns

Don't wait until your ship comes in – row out to meet it

THIS CHAPTER DEALS WITH SOME of the problems that have been commonly met with in the work-based training scheme for veterinary nursing. With the evolution of the veterinary nurse scheme some of the old problems have been resolved, some have been re-discovered and new ones have arisen. There are not answers for everything but an overall common-sense approach to many of these problems provides some help.

Within the VNAC and training-practice system there should be a good line of support and assistance available on an almost daily basis from the internal verifiers to the assessors, especially during the 'early days' of setting up a training system. Unfortunately, during the introduction of NVQs this internal verification link was missing, which probably produced quite a lot of the negative feeling towards the veterinary nurse training scheme. Some of these negative·aspects have taken on almost legendary proportions, with a number of 'horror' stories still being exchanged within veterinary circles.

Communication is such a key issue in today's society and not least so for the success of the workplace training scheme for veterinary nurses. Each training practice now has an internal verifier who can guide and support the practice and the assessor, and it is so important that this service is used. On a higher level, internal verifiers can consult the external verifiers at the RCVS for those really tricky and more unusual problems.

Workplace problems and some ideas for solutions

Providing the veterinary practice meets the basic physical requirements for training as set by the RCVS the outstanding problems are without doubt all human in origin! Training in the workplace needs to be well managed – a skill that requires constant practice to perfect.

Time

1 Lack of time

This returns us to the problem of planning. Specific time needs to be set aside for both the assessor and the trainee together. If the training practice is committed to training then time must be allocated on a regular basis, away from the busy environment of the 'shop floor', to enable both the student and the

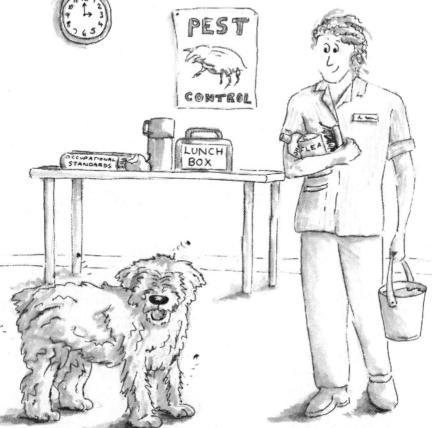

assessor to fulfil their roles. This time need not be excessive, as long as it available regularly. An hour or even 40 minutes set aside on a regular basis will be sufficient.

Regular meetings, even if only held once a fortnight, can be more economical in the long term than a snatched half hour here and there. The problems caused by lack of time can be very de-motivating to both the student and the assessor. If the assessor is fed up and de-motivated what chance does the student have? If the training practice has made a commitment to training then this commitment should be honoured.

There will always be the cry of 'too busy this week'; we have all been there. Would any practice consider treating their clients in such a way? Surely not, especially if they were working to the service ethic of the 'bonded' client who will return on a regular basis to boost the practice income. Should the practice perhaps be working to an internal ethic of the 'bonded' employee? Having spent time and effort on training an employee, the employer could hope for some stability within the 'team'. The problem of time is quite clearly a management one and as such needs to be brought to the attention of the practice principal, or whoever is ultimately responsible for the running of the practice.

Tutorial and planning sessions need to be recorded by the student and the training practice, as evidence of regular activity is expected to be provided with the completed portfolio. If problems arise these will be picked up by the internal verifier. Time management is an important part of the training practice's responsibilities and, unfortunately, this talent often seems to take a lifetime to perfect.

2   Poor use of time

Perhaps the problem with time may be that it is given, but it is not used wisely by the assessor or student. Again as before, good management is the key here. Plan ahead and be prepared to be flexible. Ensure that all log sheets are ready for assessment, that the copy of the occupational standards is at hand etc. If an assessment is to take place, ensure all staff are aware of it, especially if it might affect their working schedule. Get organized!

Economical use of evidence is another good way to help with time restrictions. Ensure that as much cross-referencing between units is carried out as is possible. For example, if possible use a medical case to meet the requirements for a fluid-therapy log sheet – there is even a possibility of a laboratory log sheet there too. Be inventive – it can be rather a challenge and quite fun. Check the detail that some students use to complete their log sheets. If the nursing of the case has been directly observed, it should not be necessary to write extra pages outside the boxes already set out on the logs. Save time if you can – it is a precious commodity for everyone.

3   Time for teaching

The following points offer some simple strategies to help learning in the clinical setting using naturally occurring material, thus making excellent use of time and opportunity.

Case discussion

Discuss a patient's case details, nursing-care plans and the details that have been explained to the owner. This helps the trainee feel part of the team and involved with patient care. This type of discussion naturally happens in most veterinary practices at staff change-over time, particularly when the staff working in the hospital environment have to 'brief' the take-over staff.

Perhaps in some practice situations it would be appropriate for the vet in charge of the case to discuss the diagnosis and care plan with the student nurse. By encouraging all members of the veterinary team to communicate regarding patient care, ideas and concepts are shared at all levels for the benefit of all, not just the student nurse.

Reflection

Take a few minutes to debrief. For example, this may be following a complicated surgical procedure – a splenectomy maybe. How did the operation go? Was the support for the patient adequate in terms of medication, analgesia, fluid therapy and anaesthesia? What type of aftercare will this patient require? Invariably, everyone has experienced this type of conversation – sometimes carried out informally over a cup of tea.

The nursing team plays a vital role in the nursing care of such a case and that team will undoubtedly include a student veterinary nurse. What a fantastic learning opportunity is presented with little or no effort. However, it is important that the veterinary team remember their secondary role as a training practice and that they look to include their trainees during these 'debriefing' sessions, however informal they may seem.

Facilitating rather than teaching

Sometimes our own personal experiences in education and learning act as a barrier to our own extended learning and, unfortunately, as a barrier to the learning experiences of others. It can be difficult not to adopt the attitude of 'this is the way we did it in my day and we had no problems'.

Many of us have had what may be considered a fairly old-fashioned education, with our teachers taking the traditional role of imparting as much information as quickly and efficiently as possible. The analogy of students as empty teacups waiting to be filled from the teapot is often used to illustrate this type of teaching. It can be argued that this type of education is very limited, as invariably you will only get back what has been put in.

Modern teaching and training is more concerned with the activity and process of learning. The role of the teacher becomes that of the facilitator, working to assist the student in actively engaging with topics and subjects to find out for themselves the how and why of things. This type of learning aims to give the individual a deeper and longer-lasting understanding and also develops the ability and necessary skills for learning, so that it can continue beyond the limits of one qualification. NVQs have been designed to use facilitators, rather than traditional teachers, within the workplace. Part of the secret with NVQs and work-based training is to recognise everyday working situations in terms of their value for training and learning opportunities, and to maximise their potential for the student.

Motivation

Many assessors have found themselves in the difficult and frustrating role of motivator. Motivation, or rather the lack of it, can be a huge problem for the student and assessor alike. Unfortunately, de-motivation is like a very nasty bout of flu – very infectious and debilitating. Therefore preventative medicine is often easier than the cure.

Generally, individuals are motivated by needs. Your trainee veterinary nurses are no different. Their training needs in the workplace are to collect evidence and to practice skills that will enable them to finally achieve their chosen qualification. They are looking for professional autonomy and responsibility within the veterinary team.

Goals, targets and feedback

It is important in a learning situation to set goals and targets. These targets need to be realistic and achievable. This is where the planning aspect of NVQs comes into play. The long-term goal for the student veterinary nurse is the completion of the portfolio as well as passing the multiple-choice question (MCQ) exam papers.

Looking at the portfolio as a whole is a daunting exercise. However, if it is broken down to bite-size chunks for shorter-term achievement, progress can be made. This is where the assessor can guide and support the student in identifying short-term goals. Individuals need to have a degree of confidence in their own abilities in order to achieve and move on to the next task. It is so important for the assessor to understand the importance and significance of feedback to the student.

The skill is to give constructive feedback on completed log sheets and only reject them if necessary. If the student's work is that poor, it may mean that they have to produce extra logs as evidence of their practical skills to meet the standards. For a new student who is perhaps having difficulty with the presentation of log sheets, it may be worth agreeing to complete a couple of practice logs that can be discussed at length.

Tracking sheets are provided to record progress made to meet the completion of the portfolio as a whole. Regular review meetings with students to discuss progress and to plan the next target can form an important part of the motivational process. Planning with the assessor also permits the students to 'take charge' and to be responsible for their own learning, a highly motivational factor for some individuals.

Motivation can also be learnt through the system of rewards. The portfolio at both levels is quite a large undertaking and it is very necessary to break it down into bite-size chunks. Most individuals will lose interest if the task set is too daunting, yet small sections can bring their own reward and pleasure as a response to successful achievement. This pleasure can work to stimulate further learning. Unfortunately for some, rewards may need to take the form of rather more material things, such as chocolate or doughnuts – leading to a rather costly exercise.

Confidence

Lack of confidence in their own abilities can be a huge de-motivating problem for students. This may be simply adjusted by increased praise for tasks successfully completed, or it may indicate a need to backtrack a couple of paces to reinforce some particular aspect of their training, double-checking their skills and understanding before progressing to the next stage.

Personalities

A clash of personality between the student and the assessor or the tutor may cause problems with progress. A third party may be necessary to resolve any major differences. If personalities are a problem, it is essential that difficulties are highlighted at an early stage and dealt with in an open and sensitive manner. In the smaller practice situation the internal verifier might be of assistance for this problem.

Workplace situation

The workplace situation can affect motivation. If learning a skill is linked to a time and place it is essential that the student is given sufficient access. For example, a Level 3 student who is trying to complete the radiography module needs to be working in the theatre rather than in the kennels or perhaps even in reception. This might appear to be an obvious problem but it is amazing how often this actually happens in practice. Organisation and planning are such an important feature of the duties and responsibilities of a training practice.

Security

In order to maximise the learning opportunities in the workplace any student needs to feel part of the working team. As an integral part of the working team the student is able to feel safe and secure and a positive attitude to tasks is fostered. Dissatisfaction can easily arise from inappropriate direction and supervision, inadequate working conditions and unsatisfactory working relationships within the team. Unfortunately, it is these negative factors rather than any positive factors that tend to be longer-lasting in their nature and resulting effect on the motivation and learning of students in the workplace. A training practice needs to have a positive attitude to successfully train their future team of nurses.

Organisational stress

Two psychological factors that influence an individual's learning and development are anxiety and stress. Anxiety and stress are influenced by the external environment. Working in a veterinary practice can be quite a stressful situation with the pressure of workload, working overtime for sick and holiday cover – let alone trying to master new skills and deal with theory input from the classroom. Training practices need to be aware of the external pressures that the workplace can put on their students and assessors. It is important that training practices have a full complement of appropriate staff to support the education and training of a student.

For many students and assessors there is an inherent tension between their role within the training and that of a paid employee. This tension can be acknowledged at the outset and addressed with the use of clear and agreed job descriptions. Staff rotas should be well planned with dates for college-course input, tutorials and training sessions clearly catered for. If the assessor is working without the support and understanding of the rest of the practice team, they can quickly become de-motivated themselves. Assessing can be hard work and this should be acknowledged by the training practice. Perhaps some sort of bonus payment for each portfolio completed would create a tangible value for the role of assessor.

On a more positive note

Hundreds of practices have worked hard to meet the standards required for training-practice status. Each of these practices has at least one assessor if not two. Student veterinary nurses are training in the workplace and they manage to complete their portfolios to meet the standards set by the RCVS in the occupational standards for veterinary nursing.

Many of these practices find that for the first time they have support and a framework that they can adapt to their own specific working practices for the training of new staff. Once awoken, this faith in training does not stop with the achievement of an NVQ certificate – it burgeons to support the notion of continuing professional development.

The high standard of nursing care that is being achieved by veterinary nursing students in the workplace is an excellent indicator that, despite the early problems of the system, many practices and nurses support and approve of the NVQ system for training veterinary nurses.

Student profile 6   Sandra

Sandra had real difficulty in keeping up with college work and her portfolio log sheets. She had a horse that kept her busy outside work hours. Sandra was working on Level 3 and realised that she was not going to meet the target for the exams. She met regularly with her assessor who sympathised with the problem and suggested that Sandra did not put herself forward for the summer examinations but delayed until the winter session. A new action plan was drawn up to enable the portfolio to be completed over a longer time frame.

As the currency of the evidence on the log sheets might possibly prove a problem, Sandra and her assessor developed a plan that would enable Sandra to complete the portfolio module by module. Thus if the need arose they could claim for unit certification. In this way any work that Sandra had already completed was safeguarded. Sandra actually completed the portfolio well within time for the winter exams and went on to pass her written papers and practical assessments with credit.

9

The Future

Adopt – Adapt – Improve

DESPITE ALL THE POLITICAL, EDUCATIONAL and funding issues veterinary surgeons still need veterinary nurses to support their practice of veterinary medicine. The professional ethics and culture of veterinary surgeons will no doubt continue to support the ideal of a recognised and worthwhile qualification for their nursing staff.

Veterinary nurses themselves are pushing for a true professional recognition of their qualification and their skills. A number of advanced certificates have been developed over recent years, like the diplomas in medicine and surgery. An equine Veterinary Nursing Certificate has been designed to enable those working with horses to achieve a recognised qualification. Qualified veterinary nurses are now 'listed'– offering evidence of their willingness to be accountable for their own actions. With the proposed changes to the Veterinary Surgeons Act 1966, there is a further case for regulation and accountability of veterinary nurses as para-professionals to the veterinary industry.

Shortage of nurses

In recent years there has appeared to be a shortage of qualified veterinary nurses. Some research has been carried out by Lantra (The Sector Skills Council for Environmental and Land-based Sector Training) to establish reasons for this. The results of this survey are intended to assist the government with the future planning and direction of funding for training schemes to meet this specific 'skill shortage' for veterinary nursing.

Interestingly, trainee and student nurses are not in short supply – in fact many practices do not need to advertise for potential trainees as they have a file full of letters inquiring about training positions. There always seems to be a good supply of 17 and 18-year-olds with the necessary GCSEs to enrol on the NVQ scheme. On the other hand, qualified nurses have always been a relatively rare commodity, as the jobs pages in the veterinary press confirm. There does seem to be a relatively large wastage of qualified individuals from veterinary practice and the following factors contribute to this.

❑ Being a particularly female-orientated profession certain wastage is bound to occur (sorry, not politically correct at all). Many nurses have left veterinary practice to start a family and found it difficult to return, either from the point of view of financing childcare or the hours of work. However, there are quite a few more part-time nurses in practice these days. As changes are made to working hours in relation to out-of-hours services, a few more veterinary nurses may be able to return to the workplace.

❑ Financial rewards are not high for veterinary nurses and in today's consumer society money can be a major issue. For some the need for a home, car and independence will mean a very necessary career change and a move to pastures new. Many nurses do not take this decision lightly but as 'needs must'. Any small business faces financial constraints on its wage structure, and the veterinary business is no exception. Perhaps, as the Veterinary Surgeons Act changes, veterinary surgeons will be more willing to consider using their nursing staff in different ways to generate more income for the business, thus supporting an improved pay structure.

Whatever the reasons for shortages of qualified staff, training veterinary nurses is an important responsibility for the veterinary profession. If this responsibility is not taken on by individual practices then it is inevitable that educational establishments, particularly those in higher education, may become a controlling influence. Will vet nurses be trained in school and then arrive ready educated, but with no really useful practical experience, three to four years later?

Lessons to be learnt?

The closest relations to veterinary medicine are found in human medicine. In recent years, human medical nursing has undergone changes in its training framework. The most notable was the introduction of the nursing degree, with all its inherent problems of combining academic achievement with essential and useful clinical skills. A particular problem with changes in nurse education was ensuring that each individual, although academically able, was also 'fit for practice'.

Many other professions are facing the same problems as they find graduates are unprepared for the realities of the workplace. Work is going on even within the veterinary surgeons' qualification to ensure the achievement of standard 'competences' for practical skills in the workplace. There is always that inherent tension between training and education.

Veterinary nursing is facing the same dilemmas and problems except that its training locations are not large NHS hospitals but small independent businesses. Despite government funding, finance can be a cause for concern both to the training practice and to the student.

Unfortunately, veterinary nurses, even if they choose to follow a degree course, will not be able to expect financial returns on a par with their human-nursing counterparts. How will nurses trained in HE establishments really be 'fit for practice'? Is veterinary nursing, in its rush for academic standing and all the anticipated rewards that brings, creating further unnecessary tensions between education and training?

The traditional or apprentice route is still the most common way to train veterinary nurses. The financial burden of this route has always rested with the training practice. The NVQ framework has given structure, quality assurance and national standards to the scheme. Unfortunately, as with any new system, the framework has taken time and effort to implement, thus adding hidden extra costs to the practices. Government funding has not been as accessible as promised and the majority of practices have received little or no financial support. The lecture course is supported by a detailed syllabus that is linked to the NVQ standards. The format of the veterinary nursing syllabus has had to be subtly changed to meet the framework for NVQs. The theoretical and examination part of an NVQ is referred to as a Vocationally Related Qualification or VRQ. All these changes are of course driven by funding issues.

Any future changes will be made to ensure that the veterinary nurse qualification continues to meet education and training funding criteria. If criteria are not met, educating veterinary nurses will cease to be a financially viable proposition for colleges. If access to funding becomes totally unavailable, the total cost of training veterinary nurses will fall to the veterinary industry.

Control of the future
The changes that have taken place over the last few years with the introduction of NVQs seemed to alienate the veterinary industry and,

at one point, the future of work-based nurse training looked very bleak. However, as the system has evolved, an uneasy acceptance of change has settled over veterinary nursing. Any further change to the work-based training scheme needs to be managed by consulting more with the veterinary industry, rather than being driven by educational and funding policies. The occupational standards for veterinary nursing will be reviewed on a regular basis along with the portfolio framework. It is important that the 'industry' is able to guide and control some of the detail to ensure that the training is still relevant to the needs of veterinary practice. Training practices and VNACs need to ensure that changes are relevant to their aims.

The industry sector – that is, veterinary surgeons and nurses – need to take an active interest in changes that are planned. The future is only what we make of it. Some of the small print of these funding packages bears some scrutiny – the old adage of 'you only get what you pay for' is very appropriate.

Decisions concerning veterinary nursing education and training issues are made at council level at the RCVS. The Veterinary Nursing Council has been reformed and now has elected nursing members to represent the veterinary nursing profession. Politics is not everyone's cup of tea but in this enlightened age of electronic communications council members can be easily contacted in order to take forward the opinions and concerns of the electorate.

Imminent change

Modern Apprenticeship schemes are the next to bring change. Remembering that colleges need to tap into all forms of possible funding by providing relevant courses, Modern Apprenticeships are a well-established work-based scheme with VRQs (Vocationally Related Qualifications) delivering the knowledge element. VRQs, combined with NVQs, are the first stage in meeting criteria for a Modern Apprenticeship work-based scheme. Subtle changes have already started to take place within the college-based courses and will probably pass unnoticed by the veterinary practices. However, before tying into a new funding scheme for student employees, it is worth reading the small print of any contract, no matter how attractive the financial support package. Everything has a price.

Whatever changes occur in the immediate future, it is important that the veterinary nurse profession continues to attract the right calibre of students who can be supported by an appropriate and successful training scheme. After all, the whole point of this exercise is the acquisition of qualified veterinary nurses to support veterinary services. A veterinary nurse needs

❏ a good basic level of education
❏ a willingness to work hard in a practical environment
❏ the ability to work as part of a team
❏ a desire , above all, to work with both animals and people.

Veterinary nursing is a very practical skill and while it does have a theoretical and academic side, the actual application is of paramount importance to the veterinary business and, of course, essential for good patient care.

A good training scheme should aim to

remove the imaginary boundaries between expertise and compassionate nursing care.

Surely this accurately reflects the work-based training scheme that is currently developing our veterinary nurses. Great care needs to be taken that we do not lose it.

Veterinary nurse: *a professional person trained in the practical application of the science and art of nursing animals under the care of a veterinary surgeon.*

Student profile 7 Judith

The fact that veterinary nursing is an NVQ enabled Judith to complete her qualification unit by unit. Judith unfortunately was diagnosed with a serious illness right at the end of her Level 2 studies. She was going to be off work for the next six months at least.

All the hard work that she had done for her portfolio was not lost as, with advice and support from the internal verifier, Judith was able to claim for seven of the eight units that make up Level 2. This meant that once Judith was fit enough to return to work she could complete the missing unit and continue with her studies to achieve Level 2 at the earliest opportunity.

Judith returned to health and completed her Level 2 NVQ. She is now studying hard for her final exams, having completed her Level 3 portfolio ahead of schedule. She has found that despite her illness she is only 12 months behind her original classmates.

Useful information

Further Reading
British Veterinary Nursing Association *Veterinary Nursing – The first twenty-five years* (BVNA 1986)

Carole Downie and Philip Basford (editors) *Teaching and assessing in clinical practice* (University of Greenwich 2000)

Ian Reece and Stephen Walker *Teaching, training and learning* (Business Education 2000)

Malcolm Tight *Key Concepts in Adult Education and Training* (Routledge 1996)

RCVS *Veterinary Nurse Training Scheme – Portfolio*

Lantra *Veterinary Nursing National Occupational Standards and Qualification Structures for NVQ Levels 2 and 3* (Lantra 2002)

Useful addresses
British Veterinary Nursing Association
Suite 11 Shenval House
South Road
Harlow
Essex CM20 2BD
Telephone   01279 450567
Fax   01279 420866
Email   bvna@bvnaoffice.plus.com

Lantra
Lantra House
Stoneleigh Park
Coventry CV8 2LG
Email   connect@lantra.co.uk
Web site   www.lantra.co.uk

RCVS
Veterinary Nursing Department
Belgravia House
62–64 Horseferry Road
London SW1P 2AF
Telephone   020 7202 0756
Email   vetnursing@rcvs.org.uk
Web site   www.rcvs.org.uk

Bottle Green Training
Unit 5 Station Yard
Station Road
Melbourne
Derbyshire DE73 1BQ
Telephone   01332 862444
Fax   01332 865165
Email   training@bgt.org.uk

Appendix 1

Veterinary Nursing NVQ Awards Units and Elements at Levels 2 & 3

LEVEL 2
The candidate must achieve all of the eight mandatory units
MANDATORY UNITS

Unit CU2	Monitor and maintain health and safety
Element CU2.1	Monitor and maintain health, safety and security in the workplace
Element CU2.2	Maintain good standards of health and safety for self and others

Unit CU5	Develop personal performance and maintain working relationships
Element CU5.1	Maintain and develop personal performance
Element CU5.2	Establish and maintain working relationships with others

Unit VN1	Carry out veterinary reception duties
Element VN1.1	Make appointments for clients and their animals
Element VN1.2	Receive clients and their animals for appointments
Element VN1.3	Process payments for veterinary services
Element VN1.4	Maintain examination rooms for use

Unit VN2	Prepare for, and assist with, medical procedures and investigations
Element VN2.1	Prepare clinical environments, equipment and materials
Element VN2.2	Prepare animals for medical procedures and investigations

Element VN2.3	Assist qualified veterinary staff during medical procedures and investigations

Unit VN3	Provide nursing care to animals
Element VN3.1	Administer medication to animals
Element VN3.2	Administer basic nursing care to animals
Element VN3.3	Administer emergency first aid to animals

Unit VN4	Care for animals in accommodation
Element VN4.1	Prepare accommodation for animals
Element VN4.2	Monitor the condition of animals in accommodation
Element VN4.3	Clean accommodation to maintain the health and safety of animals

Unit VN5	Support clients in caring for animals
Element VN5.1	Support clients during the provision of veterinary services
Element VN5.2	Advise clients on the care of animals
Element VN5.3	Demonstrate the care of animals
Element VN5.4	Provide veterinary materials to clients

Unit VN6	Admit and discharge animals
Element VN6.1	Admit animals for care
Element VN6.2	Communicate with clients regarding the progress of in-patients
Element VN6.3	Discharge animals from care

LEVEL 3

The candidate must achieve all of the seven mandatory units
MANDATORY UNITS

Unit VN7	Perform laboratory diagnostic tests
Element VN7.1	Prepare diagnostic test equipment and materials
Element VN7.2	Prepare animals for diagnostic tests
Element VN7.3	Collect and preserve samples for diagnostic tests
Element VN7.4	Carry out diagnostic tests and communicate the results

Unit VN8	Administer veterinary medical nursing to animals
Element VN8.1	Calculate and administer fluid therapy to animals
Element VN8.2	Administer specialised medical nursing and treatments to animals
Element VN8.3	Administer intensive nursing care

Unit VN9	Prepare for diagnostic imaging techniques and conduct radiography on animals
Element VN9.1	Prepare diagnostic imaging equipment and materials
Element VN9.2	Prepare animals for diagnostic imaging techniques
Element VN9.3	Conduct, and provide the results of, radiography on animals

Unit VN10	Prepare for veterinary surgical procedures
Element VN 10.1	Prepare surgical environments for veterinary surgical procedures
Element VN 10.2	Select and prepare veterinary surgical equipment and materials
Element VN 10.3	Prepare animals for veterinary surgical procedures

Unit VN 11	Assist the veterinary surgeon during surgical procedures
Element VN 11.1	Assist the veterinary surgeon during surgical procedures by providing equipment and materials
Element VN 11.2	Assist the veterinary surgeon to perform surgical procedures on animals
Element VN 11.3	Monitor and assist the recovery of animals after surgical procedures

Unit VN12	Assist the provision of anaesthetics to animals
Element VN 12.1	Prepare anaesthetic equipment and materials
Element VN 12.2	Prepare animals for anaesthesia

| Element VN 12.3 | Assist in administering and maintaining anaesthetics to animals |
| Element VN 12.4 | Assist in the recovery of animals following anaesthesia |

Unit VN13	Manage the availability of resources for the treatment and care of animals
Element VN 13.1	Manage the supply of veterinary materials
Element VN 13.2	Manage the availability of equipment for use in the veterinary practice

Appendix 2
Veterinary Nursing Approved Centres March 2004

Southern Region

Abbeydale – Vetlink Veterinary Training Ltd
Ashcott   Bridgwater TA7 9QP   nursing@vetlink.co.uk

Canterbury College
Canterbury   CT1 3AJ   www.cant-col.ac.uk

Cerberus Training and Consultancy
Henley-on-Thames   RG9 3ES   t: 01491 414113

Charter Veterinary Hospital Group
Ilfracombe   EX34 8NZ   mullacott@vetmagic.net

Chichester College, Brinsbury Campus
Pulborough   RH20 1DL   www.brinsbury.ac.uk

Earls Hall Veterinary Hospital
Westcliff-on-Sea   SS0 0NN   t: 01702 322222

Hadlow College
Tonbridge   TN11 0AL   t: 01732 850551

Kynoch and Partners Veterinary Surgeons
Crowthorne   RG45 6NE   t: 01344 774314

Lynwood School of Veterinary Nursing
Wimborne   BH21 1RQ   t: 01202 882101

Medivet
Watford   WD24 7UY   t: 01923 470000

MYF Training
Aldershot   GU11 1LZ   MYF.training@virgin.net

Plumpton College
Lewes   BN7 3AE   www.plumpton.ac.uk

RSPCA HQ
Horsham   RH13 7WN   t: 0870 7540365

Seadown Veterinary Hospital
Hythe   SO45 3NG   vets@seadown.co.uk

Sparsholt College
Winchester   SO21 2NF   www.sparsholt.ac.uk

Writtle College
Chelmsford   CM1 3RR   www.writtle.ac.uk

Scotland, Northern England and Northern Ireland

AC Training
Wigan	WN5 0PR	actraining77@cs.com

Barony College
Dumfries	DG1 3NE	www.barony.ac.uk

Beech House Veterinary Centre
Warrington	WA4 6QP	t: 01925 445500

Blacup Training
Brighouse	HD6 1BL	stephen.place@blacuptraining.co.uk

University of Edinburgh Royal (Dick) School of Veterinary Studies
Edinburgh	EH9 1QH	www.ed.ac.uk

Edinburgh's Telford College
Edinburgh	EH4 2NZ	www.telford.ac.uk

Gatehouse Veterinary Hospital
Bradford	BD15 7AA	t: 01274 480031

Greenmount College
Antrim	BT41 4PU	t: 02894 426700

Myerscough College
Preston	PR3 0RY	www.myerscough.ac.uk

North Highland College
Thurso	KW14 7EE	www.thurso.uhi.ac.uk

Northumbria School of Veterinary Nursing
Blyth	NE24 3AG	enquiries@nsvn.co.uk

Western, Central England and Wales

Bottle Green Training Ltd
Melbourne Derbyshire DE73 1BQ		training@bgt.org.uk

Croft Veterinary Clinic
Newcastle-under-Lyme ST5 0SN		t: 01728 711800

Hartpury College
Gloucestershire	GL19 3BE	www.hartpury.ac.uk

Larkmead Veterinary Group
Cholsey	OX10 9PA	t: 01491 651479

L.I.T.E Ltd
St Helens	WA10 1BA	nvqanimal@aol.com

Moulton College
Northampton	NN3 7RR	www.moulton.ac.uk

Norton Radstock College
Bristol	BS31 1TL	www.nortcol.ac.uk

Pershore Group of Colleges
Pershore	WR10 3JP	www.pershore.ac.uk

Rodbaston College
Penkridge	ST19 5PH	www.rodbaston.ac.uk

Rowe Veterinary Group
    Wotton-under-Edge   GL12 7PP   t: 01453 843295
University of Bristol Veterinary Nursing Unit
    Langford   BS40 5DU   s.f.badger@bristol.ac.uk
Warwickshire College
    Morton Morrell   CV35 9BL   www.warkscol.ac.uk

South Eastern, Central England and West Country

Abbey Veterinary Centre
    Grimsby   DN34 4TA   t: 01472 347054
Berkshire College of Agriculture
    Maidenhead   SL6 6QR   www.bca.ac.uk
Bicton College
    Budleigh Salterton EX9 7BY   www.bicton.ac.uk
College of Animal Welfare
    Godmanchester PE29 2LJ   www.caw.ac.uk
Duchy College
    Camborne   TR14 0AB   www.duchy.ac.uk/rosewarne
Easton College
    Norwich   NR9 5DX   www.easton-college.ac.uk
Julia Boness Veterinary Hospital
    Barton-le-Clay   MK45 4LP   t: 01585 612604
Parkvets
    Footscray   DA14 5HB   t: 0208 3008111
Wanstead Veterinary Hospital
    Wanstead   E11 2SY   dot@gvgwanstead.fsnet.co.uk

For more details visit http://www.rcvs.org.uk/vet_nurses/centres/list_vnac.html

Index

Pocket Practice Guides

The Veterinary Support Team Maggie Shilcock

What a pity this book was not written before I became a practice manager! ... an easy-to-read style... a must for practice libraries and for those considering joining a veterinary practice.

Penny Bredemear VN Times

...this book is a starting point for providing the veterinary support team with the training tools that they need. ...for new entrants into and the progressing members of the veterinary support team.

Christine Ann Merle DVM MB Editorial@penguin.doody.com

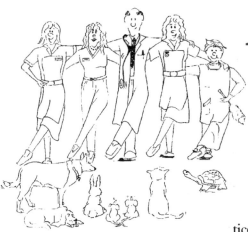

A comprehensive and practical discussion of the role of veterinary support staff and their importance to the practice—invaluable for support staff, practice managers and vets. The author, an experienced practice administrator, gives concise advice in a clear text, with plenty of diagrams and drawings.

Key topics include: how support staff create and influence the practice image, how to create co–operative support staff teams. The discussion is balanced by comments from working support staff about their jobs.

CONTENTS

Who are they and what do they do? – The practice image – Client care skills – Assertiveness and dealing with difficult clients – Support staff and money – Support staff and the office – How support staff contribute to sales and marketing – Support staff and the law – Support staff and the clinical role – Teamwork – Understanding other roles – Surviving in veterinary practice – The future

Price	£15.50 (paperback)	**Publication**	2001
Format	216 x 138 mm	**Extent**	144 pp
ISBN	1-903152-06-2	Distributed in N. America by Iowa State Press	

Premises for Vets
Designing the Veterinary Habitat
Jim Wishart DipM MCIM AMCIPD FInstSMM

An invaluable book for those thinking of embarking on modifying their practice. It is sensible and practical and its small cost will be repaid many times over during the project. Christopher J Laurence MRCVS *The Veterinary Record*

Are you making the best use of your premises and the space available? If you want to expand, what are your options? Jim Wishart, an established planner of veterinary premises, gives you the tools to decide.

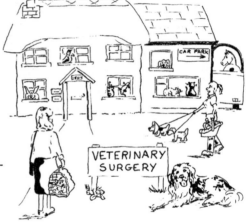

★ The extension vs. new building decision

★ Planning effective and logical work spaces and workflows

★ Finishes, furniture and flooring for optimal environments

★ Balancing clinical and health & safety requirements with cost and maintainability

★ Selecting sites and taking on the property market

★ Working with builders, architects and developers.

CONTENTS

What Do We Want to Achieve? – Thinking and Planning – Location and Site Finding – Types of Buildings and Finishes – The Design and Building Stages – **Small Animal Premises** – Front of House – In-House Services – In-Patient Treatment – **Farm Animal and Equine Facilities** – Special Requirements of Farm and Equine Work – **Turning the Key** – Promotion and Opening

£14.95 (paperback)   2002
216 x 138 mm   176 pp   1-903152-09-7